Spirituality and Aging

Spirituality and Aging

✤　✤　✤　✤

ROBERT C. ATCHLEY

The Johns Hopkins University Press
Baltimore

2 4 6 8 9 7 5 3 1

The Johns Hopkins University Press
2715 North Charles Street
Baltimore, Maryland 21218-4363
www.press.jhu.edu

Library of Congress Cataloging-in-Publication Data

Atchley, Robert C.
Spirituality and aging / Robert C. Atchley.
 p. cm.
Includes bibliographical references and index.
ISBN-13: 978-0-8018-9119-9 (hardcover : alk. paper)
ISBN-10: 0-8018-9119-1 (hardcover : alk. paper)
1. Spirituality. 2. Spiritual biography. 3. Older people—Religious life.
I. Title.
BL624.A795 2009
204.084'6—dc22   2008020970

A catalog record for this book is available from the British Library.

Illustrations on pages 58–62 are by Eugene Gregan.
Illustration on page 95 is by Melissa S. Atchley.

*Special discounts are available for bulk purchases of this book.
For more information, please contact Special Sales at 410-516-6936 or
specialsales@press.jhu.edu.*

The Johns Hopkins University Press uses environmentally friendly book
materials, including recycled text paper that is composed of at least
30 percent post-consumer waste, whenever possible. All of our book
papers are acid-free, and our jackets and covers are printed on paper
with recycled content.

To Awakened Being, with gratitude

Contents

Preface

People over 40 are primary consumers of literature, workshops, retreats, and personal growth programs concerning spirituality. "Spiritual life" is a major focus and motivator for large numbers of the people gerontologists seek to study, serve, and design programs and policies for. Yet gerontology as a field of knowledge and practice has lagged far behind its target population in understanding the importance of spirituality for aging people and developing complex concepts and language about spirituality. In this book I illustrate some ways of thinking about and discussing spirituality—what it is, why it is important, and how spirituality influences the experience of aging and vice versa. I hope to create a large conceptual/theoretical/experiential space within which readers can effectively understand, communicate, and study spirituality and aging.

The term *spirituality* refers to an inner field of human experience. It is a capacity that can grow enormously over time. Many of the most spiritually developed human beings are older men and women.

Spirituality has great potential as a vital region of continued psychological and social growth throughout adulthood. Most adults have had experiences they would label spiritual, and most see themselves as being on a spiritual journey. Perspectives on spirituality are often couched in the language and culture of various religious traditions, but since the 1960s a body of concepts, language, and theory concerning spirituality has developed in American culture that allows us to communicate, across religious boundaries, about spirituality as a topic in its own right. This language focuses on the spiritual experiences, aspirations, and resources we share as human beings.

This book is about what spirituality is, how it develops, and how it interacts with aging. It provides a conceptual map of this territory and orients the reader to spiritual development and what it means to be on a conscious spiritual journey. It will be useful to scholars who wish to study or teach about spirituality and aging and to those who wish to address the spiritual needs of aging people. I hope it will also be of use to individuals interested in spiritual growth, especially in middle and later life. The book attempts to clarify concepts and provide a theoretical framework that can advance understanding of this topic, which is so important to so many aging people.

THE ORIGINS OF THE BOOK

I believe I have an obligation to give readers an opportunity to see this book as an outgrowth of my thirty-year interest in spirituality and aging. Please bear with me here; the account is somewhat detailed and the trail may seem winding, but each part of it is important in the continuous expansion and integration of my understanding of what spirituality is and how it relates to aging.

I have been interested in spiritual experience since I was a young boy, but my conscious spiritual journey did not begin until the mid-1970s, when I was about 35. At that time I began a systematic study of the literature in the field of spirituality, and I found this field rich in perspectives and insights but also confusing. At this point I was about ten years into my academic career teaching gerontology, doing gerontology research, and writing articles, monographs, and textbooks in gerontology.

I was struck by the extent to which research and teaching about adult development and aging had ignored spiritual concerns. Many people I encountered in my research and on my personal spiritual journey were elders who had been consciously nurturing their spiritual capacities for many decades and for whom spirituality was a strong motivating force in their lives, a significant anchor for lifestyle decision making, and an important resource in coping with what life brought.

By 1980, I had collected enough scholarly material on spiritual development to begin to include this subject in my graduate course on adult psychosocial development. I also began to include questions on spirituality in my twenty-year longitudinal study of aging and adaptation (Atchley 1999). Steadily, for more than a decade, I developed a fluency with the emerging nonreligious vocabulary on spirituality, because I saw this language as a key for communicating about spirituality while avoiding the experience of division that often accompanies the use of religious concepts and language about spirituality in interfaith or secular settings.

In 1992, I attended a conference called "Conscious Aging," which was sponsored by the Omega Institute and featured speakers such as Ram Dass and

Rabbi Zalman Schachter-Shalomi, from the world of spiritual awakening and development, and Maggie Kuhn, Rick Moody, and Thomas Cole, from the world of gerontology. I was invited by the Omega staff to be part of a think tank, "The Future of Conscious Aging," in the summer of 1995.[1] As a concept, conscious aging did not mean being aware of one's aging; it meant aging in a spiritually awakened state.

In that time period I also began publishing my ideas about spirituality and spiritual development. I published articles on spiritual development and wisdom (Atchley 1993) and the everyday nature of spiritual development in later life (Atchley 1997a), and I added material on the nature of spirituality and spiritual development and its relationship to aging in the eighth edition of my gerontology textbook, *Social Forces and Aging* (Atchley 1997b). I also published the results of my longitudinal study, which showed that the importance of spiritual development increased over time (Atchley 1999). This study is mentioned at several points in this book.

I have adapted three previously published articles for this volume: "The Influence of Spiritual Beliefs and Practices on the Relation between Time and Aging" (Atchley 2001), which appears as Chapter 7; "Becoming a Spiritual Elder" (Atchley 2003), which is part of Chapter 4; and "Continuity, Spiritual Growth, and Coping in Later Adulthood" (Atchley 2006), which is Chapter 6.

I mention this background to make three points: (1) I have been working in the field of aging for forty years and the field of spirituality and spiritual development for thirty years; (2) I have expended much effort researching, talking with people, contemplating, and writing about spirituality and aging; and (3) I have sought feedback on my work from others who have also been writing on spirituality—from students, from professionals working in the field of aging, and from members of the general public who are interested in the subject of spirituality and aging.

I did not develop my ideas and language about spirituality and aging sitting in an "ivory tower." I developed them using an open-feedback system in which I read and contemplated, interviewed aging people, listened to sages, observed aging people in a variety of environments, meditated, wrote summaries and tentative conclusions, took those imperfect insights out into the field and got feedback (by no means uniformly positive), and went back to the drawing board over and over again. I have readjusted my frames of reference and information base many times over the course of this journey. A main challenge is to stay open to discovery. The more I can keep my attachments to my own ideas loose, the greater the possibility for new clarity to appear.

This book is an attempt to share what I have learned as of 2008. No doubt I have much more to learn, but I have a well-tested and serviceable picture of the complexity and grandeur and struggles involved in the spiritual region of human life and how this region influences aging, and vice versa.

During the period when these ideas were developing, I was myself growing older. When I began teaching and writing about spirituality, I was in my 40s, and as I put the finishing touches on this book early in 2008, I am 68. This is not a necessary qualification for understanding the subject of this book, but my personal experiences of both spirituality and aging provide me with a depth and richness of experience that I think has made me a better, more tuned-in reader, listener, and participant. Living with the concepts and language of spirituality for such a long time has affected what I perceive in texts I read, conversations I hear, and experiences I have. I am much more aware now of the layers that lie within texts and the high degree to which adequate interpretation depends on a deep background in the subject. I think it is no accident that, for centuries, philosophical and spiritual wisdom has mostly been the province of people with a lot of life experience with the subject.

THE PLAN OF THE BOOK

The Introduction provides an overview of the book and some orienting discussion of the concepts and language that are used to describe and discuss spirituality.

Part One consists of three chapters that provide basic frames of reference for our examination of spirituality and aging. Chapter 1 deals with the nature of spirituality, from its beginnings in pure being and transcendence, to the various avenues through which spiritual being manifests itself, to qualities that typify spiritual experiences, to how spirituality influences experience in many aspects of life. Chapter 2 looks at spiritual development as an evolutionary process that can occur both naturally and consciously. It considers spiritual development in the context of adult development generally and looks at ways in which spiritual development illustrates the higher possibilities of adult development. Chapter 3 focuses on spiritual identity and on the spiritual self and how it differs from the objective self, which comprises self-concept, self-ideal, and self-esteem.

Part Two focuses on two dimensions of spirituality that are especially likely to emerge and ripen in later life: becoming a sage and serving from spirit. Becoming a sage is about the development of a capacity to bring spiritual perspective to everyday issues. Chapter 4 considers ways in which people consciously and nonconsciously evolve into a type of transpersonal psychology that makes wisdom possible. Chapter 5 looks at how aging and spiritual development intersect to create opportunities for a different kind of service, a service rooted in spiritual being. It also describes how organizations might operate from principles of transpersonal sociology to match the transpersonal psychology of the organization's members.

Part Three consists of three chapters that illustrate how spirituality and spiritual development interact with other specific aspects of life. Chapter 6 looks at how continuity theory and conceptions of spiritual development can be combined to better understand how people cope with opportunities and constraints that arise in later life. Chapter 7 takes on a relatively specific topic: how spiritual beliefs and practices influence age changes in the experience of time. Chapter 8 looks at how spirituality and aging influence the experience of dying and death.

In the Conclusion, I look back over the examination of spirituality and aging, summarize and reflect on what we have discovered, and draw implications for future study, education, and practice within the field of aging.

Acknowledgments

My recent books have begun with a nudge from my wife and colleague, Sheila Atchley. Sheila is more familiar than anyone with what I am thinking about and studying, and at some point in my process Sheila will say, "I think you need to write a book about that." So it was with spirituality and aging. The positive value of Sheila's steady appreciation of my work is immeasurable.

Susan McFadden has encouraged my work on spirituality and aging since the early 1990s. She is an astute sounding board and skilled critic who appreciates what I have to say and unerringly helps me say it better. She created several opportunities for me to participate in conferences and write book chapters that prodded me into thinking more clearly about spirituality and aging. For this book, she gave me a great deal of specific feedback that helped me flesh out and organize my ideas and examples.

Harry "Rick" Moody has also been supportive. Beginning with our time together on the Omega Institute's "Conscious Aging Think Tank" in the mid-1990s, Rick and I have traveled parallel paths in the area of spirituality and aging, although we look at different scenery at times. Rick has been generous in creating opportunities for me to participate in a variety of conferences and projects in which I have learned a great deal about the subject of this book. Rick wrote a detailed critique of this book manuscript, one that challenged and helped me to clarify points and make it more accessible.

Wendy Harris, at the Johns Hopkins University Press, listened with encouragement and interest to several iterations of my ideas about a book on spirituality and aging. She has a knack for raising the right questions and issues to expand or clarify my thinking. She was helpful in organizing the book.

I also want to acknowledge and thank the many people who participated in my research studies and in several study groups I observed over the years. I thank those who attended my presentations and asked good questions, those who challenged my ideas (of these there were many), and those who allowed me into their lives for a little while so that I could ground my ideas in some semblance of reality. Without these hundreds of people, I would not have experienced directly the diversity and richness that is the field of spirituality and aging.

I have learned much from my twelve years of participation in Quaker Meetings, first in Oxford, Ohio, and later in Boulder, Colorado. The Quaker culture of inner discovery, spiritual seeking in community, and transpersonal group process has informed important aspects of my understanding of spirituality and aging. Also, wise and spiritual elders are prevalent in these communities, and they helped me identify what to look for in people who exemplify the higher stages of spiritual development.

Spirituality and Aging

Introduction

Setting the Stage

This book considers fundamental questions about the meaning of being and how it is shaped by the experience of aging. The following general questions guided my study of spirituality and aging:

— What is spirituality?
— What makes an experience "spiritual"?
— What does it mean to grow spiritually?
— How does spirituality affect identity and self?
— What is the nature of a spiritual journey?
— How does confidence and trust in a spiritual process develop?
— How does spirituality manifest itself in everyday life?
— What does it mean to build a life around spiritual concerns?
— How are these questions shaped by and how do they influence the experience of aging?[1]

First and foremost, spirituality is a region of human experience.[2] Without our own inner experience of the spiritual region of life, talk about spirituality is akin to science fiction. We can imagine what spiritual experience might be like, but that is by no means the same as having the experience. Later on, we will see that spiritual experiences have qualities that set them apart from other experiences, qualities such as wonder, compassion, or clarity. Spiritual experiences occur through a variety of avenues, such as our senses, consciousness/awareness, or thought. The spiritual region of human experience is valuable in its own right to most people, and it can also influence other aspects of life, such as human development, personal history, and personal goals.

As a viewpoint or vantage point, spirituality can take three basic forms:

intense awareness of the present, transcendence of the personal self, or a feeling of connection with all of life, the universe, a supreme being, or a great web of being. Most people grow into these perspectives in a succession or upward spiral of increasing understanding we call spiritual development or spiritual growth. Many come to recognize that these vantage points are interrelated and can reside in awareness simultaneously.

As a topic of discussion, the inner experience I am calling spirituality was called "private religion" in the early twentieth century (James 1905), and it was assumed that religion offered the major, if not the only, pathway to this type of experience. But during the 1950s it became increasingly clear that many people had spiritual experiences without benefit of religion, so calling these experiences "religious" did not make much sense.[3] There was also a trend at this time toward mistrust of institutional religion,[4] which discounted religion's authority in the area of inner experience. "You may well tell me what I *ought* to think, but you can't tell me what I *do* think."

At about that same time, there was a revival of the ancient idea that we all have an innate potential for spiritual experience that can be developed into a capacity.[5] This idea, combined with the idea that we exert influence over our own development, fueled an interest in spiritual development as a personal goal.[6] Thus, people began to speak about their "spiritual journey" as an intentional direction for spiritual development and to express a preference for a lifestyle that supports such a journey.

The concept of a spiritual journey refers to an individual's personal narrative about her or his spiritual life and its development, including its ups and downs. This narrative usually includes a history of experiences, actions, and insights connected with a search for spiritual meaning. Underlying the spiritual journey is an intentional process of seeking spiritual experiences, using spiritual values and insights to inform life choices, and learning from experience with this process. The spiritual journey for most people involves bringing spirituality ever more completely into consciousness and learning to be consciously aware of the spiritual aspects of most human experiences.

Spiritual journeys also involve learning to persist and be content on a journey into imperfectly known territory, where insights are always limited, no matter how profound they may seem at the time. People who have been on a spiritual journey for decades usually have developed a sense of humor about the contradictions and paradoxes they encounter, even as they use these enigmas as food for contemplation. People also learn not to force the issue. Waiting is an important spiritual practice—not "waiting for" but just waiting. In the space created by patient waiting, connection with the sacred, or "ground of being," is more likely.

Most spiritual journeys also involve elements of commitment, self-discipline, and regular spiritual practice. I will discuss these elements in detail later, but I mention them to round out the picture of spiritual journeys.

In his insightful review of social change in spiritual thought and behavior in the last half of the twentieth century, Robert Wuthnow (1998) argues that spirituality in America shifted from a religion-centered "spirituality of dwelling" toward a person-centered "spirituality of seeking" and later toward a personal "spirituality of practice." Spirituality of dwelling "emphasizes habitation: God occupies a definite place in the universe and creates a sacred space in which humans too can dwell; to inhabit sacred space is to know its territory and to feel secure" (3–4). A spirituality of dwelling emphasizes the security available from firm adherence to doctrine and worship primarily in awe-inspiring edifices and rituals. A spirituality of dwelling also emphasizes unchanging doctrine, ritual, and organizational structure. Comfort, security, and answers come from predictability.

By contrast, a spirituality of seeking emphasizes journeying and negotiation. On a journey, we never know exactly what we will confront, but we have to remain aware of our needs and pay attention to opportunities to make effective decisions. Spiritual journeying requires that an individual learn to negotiate a landscape filled with "complex and confusing meanings of spirituality" (ibid., 4). On the spiritual journey, we never have perfect maps, so we need an enduring set of questions that will allow us to discover the ground of being in that time and place. We try to "live the questions" (Rilke 2002, 21).

Wuthnow (1998) says that a spirituality of seeking is especially likely to emerge in unsettled times, and this may explain why people who came of age in the late 1950s and thereafter tended to be more receptive to and interested in a spirituality of seeking. The environment of seeking occurs in mind-boggling diversity, ranging from sparkling new megachurches, to revitalized traditional congregations, to informal Sunday-morning meetings in unused bars, to solitary journeys made mostly in silence. People seek in the kind of environment in which they feel nurtured and nourished, and most people seek the company of kindred spirits.

Wuthnow (1998) argues that most people live a life that balances dwelling and seeking. They like both the security of dwelling and the openness of seeking. He also sees an emerging practice-oriented spirituality that emphasizes a practice-oriented life, which, come what may, provides an ongoing, constant commitment to doing the hard work of nurturing spirituality. Thus, we become what we do, and returning to spiritual practice over and over again creates habits of mind and habits of being that come to seem natural. But because these spiritual practices are most often part of an open context of spiritual seeking rather than a closed system of doctrine and ritual, these habits can become enlivening instead of stifling. Spiritual practices are things we do on a regular basis to celebrate, appreciate, nurture, and act on our experiences of presence, transcending the personal self, and connecting directly with the sacred. Many types of meditation and prayer, devotional rituals and music, inspirational reading and reflection, and movement-oriented spiritual disciplines, such as labyrinth walking, yoga, and tai chi, can be mixed and matched to support a contemplative, practice-oriented spirituality.

There are many spiritual traditions, each of which has its own unique language and concepts concerning the nature of the ultimate, the path that must be followed to experience the ultimate, how spiritual realizations are confirmed, the nature of spiritual enlightenment, and the implications of spiritual understanding for ordinary human life. Although it would be a mistake to gloss over the importance of the differences this variety produces, each of the major faith groups—Christianity, Islam, Judaism, Buddhism, Taoism, Hinduism—is rooted in the profound, direct, authentic mystical experiences of its founder(s). Moses, Jesus, Buddha, and Muhammad all are reported to have attained their spiritual messages at least initially through a profound mystical experience that happened in solitude. The contemporary surge in inner exploration may in many cases be an attempt by individuals to experience those insights for themselves, to move beyond a second-hand notion of spirituality as something that must be channeled by the clergy or other spiritual authority figures toward authentic, independent, and direct experiences of spirituality.[7] In meditation and prayer, learning to dwell in silence can play an important part in creating an inner opening for spiritual experience. Such inner explorations can take place in the context of traditional religious groups or alternative groups that take a more universalistic view of the spiritual journey. Some make their spiritual journey alone, following the inner light.

There is considerable evidence that spiritual concerns, experience, and development become increasingly important for many people in middle and later life. This evidence can be found in the narratives of individuals as well as in social science surveys (Atchley and Barusch 2004). Beginning around age 35 or 40, as age increases, so does the proportion of people who are consciously involved in an inner exploration of the meaning of their existence and their relation to the universe. Albert Winseman (2003) reported that adults age 65 or older were more than twice as likely to see themselves as spiritually committed than were adults age 45–54. Spiritually committed people are often engaged in spiritual practices that heighten the possibility of noumenous, mystical experience. In addition, those who experience transcendent, nonpersonal levels of consciousness often feel called to serve, and spiritually rooted service takes many forms.

The study of aging developed at a time when our cultural conceptions about the spiritual region of life were shifting from a religion-oriented concept rooted in scripture and traditional rituals to a personal responsibility concept based in experience, choice, and personal discipline. Most of the research on spirituality and aging has been conducted from a religion-oriented conception of spirituality. But the population of elders is increasingly made up of individuals who see themselves as having been on a personal spiritual journey of many years' duration. It is time to devise a viable framework for studying spirituality that reflects the concepts about spirituality that are being used by the people we study. I hope in this book to provide the beginnings of such a framework.

Spirituality is a popular topic in the United States at present. For example, in November 2007 the online bookseller Amazon.com listed more than 130,000 book titles having to do with spirituality. Although most authors seem comfortable writing about spirituality, only a few attempt to define it specifically.

That so many writers "talk around" the topic of spirituality rather than meet it head-on is, I think, a reflection of the nature of the spiritual region of life. Many years ago the sociologist Herbert Blumer made a useful distinction between denotative and sensitizing concepts.[8] Denotative concepts refer to an observable part of life. For example, church attendance is a denotative concept; it has a concrete referent. Sensitizing concepts, on the other hand, do not point to something specific or concrete but instead deal with qualities to be sensitive to if we want to observe or communicate about a general field or region. In my view, spirituality is a concept that sensitizes us to a region of human experience and tells us generally what to look for in that region, but no concept can tell us what specific combination of qualities and avenues of spiritual experience will be present in any given spiritual experience.

Sensitizing concepts can be discussed with our usual discursive language, but the metaphors of parables or poetic thought are often more effective, because metaphors suggest rather than direct what is to be seen. Take, for example, this poem by Rumi (Barks 1995, 36):

> Out beyond ideas . . . there is a field. I'll meet you there.
> When the soul lies down in that grass, the world is too full to talk about.
> Ideas, language, even the phrase *each other* doesn't make any sense.

Where is this field beyond thought? Whom will we meet there? If *each other* doesn't make any sense, what does? This poetic statement engages and challenges and opens us differently than analytic thought does.

Compare Rumi's poem with this discursive statement by Roger Walsh (1999, 3): "Spirituality . . . refers to *direct experience* of the sacred." Walsh's statement is meaningful, provided we know what *the sacred* is, but in my opinion it does not invite the experience it defines to the same extent that Rumi's poem does. I have found that poetry and metaphorical stories are often more effective than discursive text as stimuli for discussions of spirituality, perhaps because poetry and metaphors invite deeper unstated feelings and needs into the conversation.

If we are to see spirituality as a holistic region of human experience, then we need to employ many more methods than usual. Our empirical, conceptual, and analytical capacities must be augmented by humanistic capacities such as contemplation, rumination,[9] imagination, and intuition.

Nevertheless, we still need some basic vocabulary to begin with, and dictionary definitions are a good place to start. For example, in the *American Heritage Dictionary* (2006), *spirituality* is defined as "the state, quality, or fact of being spiritual." *Spiritual* is defined as "of, relating to, or consisting of, or having the nature of spirit." *Spirit* is defined as "one's unseen, intangible being." *Being* is defined as "existence." Thus, spirituality is rooted in our purest experience of existence, the "I Am" without words, just awareness. As experience, pure being does not require an object (I am this or I am that), and it exists prior to, and as a prerequisite for, all other experiences, including time and space. As such, spirituality in its purest form is an inner, subjective experience. Pure, nonverbal experience of being is the spiritual field within which occur the mindfulness and present-moment awareness of Buddhists, the Christ-consciousness of Christians, the witness-consciousness of Hindus, the awe so prized by Jews, and the ecstatic consciousness of Muslims.

As experience, spirituality as being may or may not be related to experience of a higher or greater or deeper power. George Gallup (2003) reported that almost a third of a national sample of adults defined spirituality without reference to a higher power. Most people consider spirituality to be related to a big picture because of the common experience that one's own being is linked to a larger web of being, an experience that one is not alone but is part of something much greater than individual existence. This experience is usually based in an intuitive form of knowing. This is where Walsh's concept of spirituality as direct experience of the sacred comes in, if *sacred* is defined as that which is considered holy, given reverence, respect, and wonder, and is derived from a divine source (adapted from the *American Heritage Dictionary* 2006). Cultural differences lead this experienced linkage between the "I Am" and the great web of being to be described or articulated in many different ways, based on language and history.

When an individual makes a shift from experiencing personal existence as a solitary being to experiencing existence as part of a larger being or web of being, then transcendence can be said to have occurred. Not all forms of transport are transcendence. For example, it is quite possible for awareness to increase markedly in intensity without making the profound shift in level of consciousness that occurs when one touches or merges with what Aldous Huxley (1944, viii) called the "immanent and transcendent Ground of all being." (Paul Tillich [1967] can be credited with introducing American culture to the concept "ground of being" as a way of conceiving of God that goes beyond the personified conceptions of God prevalent in American religion and popular culture at the time.)[10]

We usually experience spirituality not in an inner vacuum of pure existence but in the context of acting in some way, even if that action is deep contemplation while sitting relatively still. Undoubtedly, pure being is present underneath everything we do. If we are not experiencing being, how can we experience anything else?

The spiritual journey can be seen as a quest for balance between being and doing. In the process of learning to function in the social worlds into which we are born—family, work, community, society, and so on—many people become overly focused on acting within the context of socially defined positions and roles, their attention is absorbed by this social world, and they lose sight of the liberating "qualities of being" that are there also. We learn to identify with our niches, actions, and lifestyles rather than with our more fundamental being. The spiritual journey is often about learning to bring *being* back into our consciousness. People are often motivated toward this sort of journey by their feeling that something is missing from their conventional role-centered lives. For many people, learning to bring being back into consciousness introduces a healthy distance from, and perspective on, social roles and also a needed element of creativity and spontaneity to one's lived experience.

As we try to understand the interaction between spirituality and other aspects of life, we discover that these relationships are at least as complicated as everything else in our lives and may involve even more levels of consciousness and awareness than we are accustomed to dealing with. Spirituality is a difficult and complex topic only because we yearn to integrate it into how we see our lives. If we were comfortable just letting spirituality run in the subconscious background, we would not have much to do. But if our experience tells us that being consciously in touch with pure being, self-transcendence, and the ground of being enhances the quality of our life, and if we want to understand why this is so, then we are drawn to develop the concepts and theoretical linkages needed to think and study and communicate about this important topic. Also, if we want to understand how the spiritual region of life interacts with aging, we need a good map of the spiritual region.

A major goal of this book is to provide a conceptual and theoretical picture of spirituality that is much broader, deeper, higher, more interrelated, symphonic, full-spectrum, and panoramic than the narrow views used in much of the current work on spirituality and aging. It is also important to emphasize that this book looks at spirituality as a topic separate from religion. Although many people find that their religious beliefs provide an important and perhaps exclusive context for experiencing spirituality, as age increases so does the proportion of people who see spirituality in a broader context than formal or organized religion (Roof 1999; Zinnbauer et al. 1997). The difference is that, while many studies emphasize religion with a nod toward spirituality, here I emphasize spirituality with a nod toward religion. But because most religions contain language and practices intended to facilitate experiences of pure being and connection, there will inevitably be points where religion and spirituality overlap. In everyday life it may not be necessary to disentangle the two, but if we want to understand spirituality well enough to study it adequately, include it in our ideas about appropriate practice and service to elders, and avoid unnecessarily joining it and religion, we need to keep our focus on spirituality and not on religion. This is in no way a negative statement about religion, but simply a desire to stick to the subject.

I also avoid religious language as much as possible because I have found that, although it may be helpful for the in-group, it often activates a sense of intergroup division and difference. Religious language also usually implies a specific theological interpretation of spirituality. If we can find ways to base our dialogues on our *experiences* of being, self-transcendence, and the ground of being, stated in language that does not invoke religious concepts, we may be able to have conversations about spiritual experiences we share instead of about our different religious concepts.

I must also acknowledge that the words *spiritual* and *spirituality* are often met with open hostility. Interestingly, many people who are hostile toward the terms are quite able to discuss their experiences of this region of life, which suggests that their hostility is a response to specific language and the "baggage" it carries and not to the reality the language was developed to describe. Unfortunately, I have tried many alternative terms and none escapes this problem.

Finally, this book is also about how experiences of spirituality interact with experiences of adult development and aging. This begs the question of when aging begins. For our purposes, aging is assumed to begin for most people when they are in their forties. In my longitudinal study of aging and adaptation (Atchley 1999), a large majority of people said that by age 70 their inner life had increased in importance compared with when they were 50. Many people considered spirituality to be a capacity that continues to develop within a person no matter what happens with aging. Also, spirituality was cited by many as an important resource for coping with the challenges of aging. A big portion of this book concerns the evolutionary processes through which people develop spiritually.

My goal is to provide a systematic treatment of spirituality as a subject in its own right and to expand the view of spirituality to match the richness and complexity that it has in the everyday worlds of many middle-aged and older people.

With this overview of the approach used in this book, we can proceed now to Part I, which explores the nature of spirituality, how spirituality develops, and the inter-relationship of spirituality with identity and self.

Basic Frames of Reference

CHAPTER ONE

The Nature of Spiritual Experience

There is no doubt that many people have experiences they label *spiritual.* Spirituality can be seen as the capacity to perceive experiences as spiritual. But what qualifies an experience to be called spiritual? What criteria do people use? Is spiritual experience something separate from "ordinary" experience or does *spiritual* refer to a quality that can accompany many types of experiences? This chapter develops a framework for addressing these questions.

Serious discussion of spirituality as an important aspect of human nature, the identification of pathways for inner spiritual growth and development, and reports of direct spiritual experiences have been part of the written cultural legacy of humanity for at least five thousand years (Radhakrishnan 1989). As mentioned earlier, I am using *spirituality* to refer to an inner, experiential region of human life. Spiritual experience can occur at many levels: physical, emotional, cognitive, and transcendent. Spirituality is a quality that can infuse experience in a wide variety of settings. Spiritual experience can be both transcendent and immanent: It can be both an experience of transcending worldly concerns as well as an intense present-moment perception that the ground of all being permeates things. The essence of fully developed spirituality is an intense aliveness and deep sense of understanding that one intuitively comprehends as having come from a direct, internal link with that mysterious principle that connects all aspects of the universe. As fully awakened spiritual beings, we feel our interconnectedness.

In most spiritual traditions, mysticism lies at the heart of spirituality. *Mysticism* refers to transcendent, contemplative experiences that enhance spiritual understanding. Mystical experiences can occur during intentional practices designed to create conditions conducive to transcendent experiences, such as Zen meditation, Christian centering prayer, or Sufi dance. Mystical experiences can also occur in the process of living a lifestyle that is conducive to transcendent experiences, as in contemplative gardening. In either case, contemplative or transcendent knowing may be associated with spiritual experience.

Transcendence refers to contemplative knowing that occurs outside the boundaries of verbal thought (Wilber 2001). Although transcendence can refer to increasingly abstract thought (Pascual-Leone 1990), contemplative transcendence involves transcending thought itself. Mystical experiences of transcendence can be brought into thought, but they do not originate in thought or sensory perception.

Organized religions are social groups or social institutions that have both theological and behavioral doctrines, ministerial or clerical authority, and ritualized social worship. The size, scope, and history of religious organizations varies enormously. Of course, individual members can and do internalize both the theological beliefs and behavioral prescriptions and proscriptions associated with their organized religion. Individuals often find their deepest spiritual experiences in the context of their religion. But individuals also often have their own unique interpretations of the tenets of their religion.

The relation of religion and spirituality is in the eye of the beholder. Many people use *religion* and *spirituality* as synonyms and see no difference between the two terms. Others use *religion* to refer to a sociocultural program for developing spiritually and for bringing spiritual realizations into everyday life, and they use *spirituality* to refer to the inner experiences that arise from trying to put such programs into practice. Most people see *spirituality* as the broader term, one that includes a greater variety of experiences than they would include in the term *religion*. Some people attach little or no importance to organized religion but at the same time see themselves as spiritual persons.

Brian Zinnbauer and colleagues (1997) surveyed 346 men and women from diverse groups, ranging from mental health workers to traditional religious denomination members to conservative Christians, concerning their interpretation of the terms *spirituality* and *religiousness*. Concerning which was the broader term, 38.8 percent saw *spirituality* as broader and 10.2 percent saw *religiousness* as broader (table 1).

A large majority (74%) saw themselves as both spiritual and religious, and 19 percent saw themselves as spiritual but not religious. Only 4 percent saw themselves as religious but not spiritual, and 3 percent saw themselves as nei-

TABLE 1
The Relation of Spirituality and Religiousness

Response	Percentage
Spirituality and religiousness overlap but are not the same concept	41.7
Spirituality is the broader term	38.8
Religiousness is the broader term	10.2
Spirituality and religiousness do not overlap	6.7
Spirituality and religiousness overlap completely	2.6

Source: Adapted from Zinnbauer et al., 1997.
  Note: N = 346

ther. Another way of expressing these findings is that 93 percent saw themselves as spiritual and 78 percent saw themselves as religious (table 2).

George Gallup (2003) reported that 75 percent of respondents to a 1999 Gallup Poll saw spirituality as "personal and individual" rather than as involving "organized religion and church doctrine."

These findings support the separation of spirituality and religiousness within the study of subjective aspects of the region of life involving perceptions and expressions of the sacred.

As a topic in the study of aging, spirituality has mostly been seen as a part of religion, despite many surveys showing that many people consider themselves to be spiritual but not religious. Harold Koenig (2001, 505), after his thorough review of the literature on spirituality, wrote that "spirituality is a broader, more inclusive term than religiosity. Many measures of spirituality that exist today, however, measure simply religiosity."

As Robert Wuthnow (1998) pointed out, since the 1950s there has been a growing tendency to use *spiritual* to refer to inner experiences and *religious* to refer to external experiences connected with organized religion. Many authors who grew up with a religion-centered approach to inner spiritual experiences prefer to use *religious* to refer to both types of experience (Pargament 1997; Roof 1999; Smith 2001). They try to reduce spirituality to religion by assuming that any inner experience of the ground of being is religious, even if the person having the experience is unchurched or lacking in religious background. Reporting on Gallup Polls conducted annually from 1978 to 1998, Michael Lindsay (2000) found that the percentage of adult Americans identified as "unchurched"—no membership in a religious community and no church attendance in the past six months—remained steady at 41–44 percent throughout the twenty-year period. More to the point, I think, is that words

TABLE 2
Identification with Spirituality and Religiousness

Response	Percentage
I am spiritual and religious	74
I am spiritual but not religious	19
I am religious but not spiritual	4
I am neither spiritual nor religious	3

Source: Adapted from Zinnbauer et al., 1997.
   Note: $N = 346$

mean what a person takes them to mean, not what authority figures want them to mean. In today's world, *spiritual* is seen by a majority of people to be a broader term than *religious* and to refer to an inside-out personal learning process rather than an outside-in socialization process (Roof 1999).

To begin to grasp the diversity of experiences that qualify as spiritual, I began about ten years ago to ask people to describe an experience that they would label spiritual. I have asked this question of hundreds of people, mostly middle-aged and older. Here is a sampling of responses, selected for their diversity.

Some people provided an overview.

As I tried to think about your question, I began to wonder if any experiences are *not* spiritual. If being spiritual is part of our nature, maybe even the central part, which I believe it is, then as long as we are being, there is a spiritual element. Whether we are aware of it is another thing.

Man, age 92

＃

I wouldn't describe any experience as spiritual. That word has never had much personal meaning for me. I have had experiences that were inspiring, even transcendent, and I don't know what to call them as a category.

Man, age 80

＃

Life is more and more spiritual all the time. I have an ongoing experience of being part of a network. It is the backdrop to everything. Sometimes it is faint, almost not there, when I deal with the logistics of everything that I am part of and that is part of me. This "tuning in" has become easier since I moved out of the city.   *Woman, age 52*

Some found spiritual experiences in religious contexts.

> I went with some friends to a revival meeting to hear a well-known preacher. He was a plain little man who didn't look well. He greeted each of us at the door, and I could smell his bad breath. A few minutes later he stepped up onto a small stage and began to speak about the Holy Spirit. His air of frailty was gone and he seemed strong and energetic. The cadence of his gravelly voice was hypnotic, like he was inviting the Holy Spirit. Suddenly, I felt myself expand inside and that expanse was filled with the warmth and love of the Holy Spirit.   *Woman, age 46*

Others found spiritual experience in nature.

> Last year my husband and I traveled to the Grand Canyon for the first time. As I stood on the South Rim and looked into the great expanse of the canyon, I was overcome by the massive *stillness* of the giant rock formations bearing scars from thousands of years of wind and water. Just resting with the canyon for a few minutes evoked that stillness in me. It was a tremendous sense of peace and release. Just thinking about it now brings that feeling back.   *Woman, age 67*

Some found spiritual experience in relating with others.

> When I'm with a group of friends, catching up on each other's lives, I often am aware that we are connected by something holy and that holy connection is what we are really celebrating through all our energetic talking.   *Woman, age 49*

Others found spiritual experience in doing service.

> Periodically I go with a group of friends to our local shelter for the homeless to prepare the evening meal. The people who come through the food line are an amazing mixture. Most are in their 30s and 40s and many have obvious mental problems of one kind or another. Most show the wear and tear of living on the streets. When I first started doing this, I found it difficult to be around that much suffering all in one place. The discomfort I felt made me want to close down, to harden my heart. But I knew somehow that I needed to do just the opposite, to summon all the reserves of love I could find and stand there with a heart open to the suffering. Through this I was able to gently connect spiritually with the people being served and realize that we are all being served.   *Woman, age 43*

For some, spiritual experience was primarily sensory.

> Feeling the hot water on my hands, hearing the sounds of sloshing water, and seeing the light reflected off the wet dishes are spiritual to me.
>
> *Woman, age 80*

Others found spiritual experience as part of their work.

> I work as a massage therapist, and I often work with people who are vulnerable. I was trained to approach my clients with nonjudgmental acceptance and attentiveness. It feels to me that when people are on my massage table, they are exposing themselves in more ways than one, in that they are trusting me with their self-conscious and imperfect selves, not just bodily. As I am touching these people, I am often meeting them at a much deeper level than their skin. I experience more than just meeting spirit to spirit or soul to soul; the experience feels more like I am, in fact, not separate from this person but that we are part of a whole.
>
> *Woman, age 66*

From the diversity of these responses, we can see that spiritual experience is a big category indeed. Spiritual experience can occur in many different types of environment and under a wide variety of circumstances. Even within the same person, there are usually many avenues for having experiences labeled spiritual. Imagine what would happen if I asked about spiritual history, spiritual capacity, spiritual states, spiritual practice, spiritual identity, and spiritual growth. We could expect highly individualized answers to these questions as well. Quickly we can begin to understand why in-depth study of the spiritual region of life has seldom been attempted, especially in combination with other topics, such as aging and adult development.

QUALITIES PRESENT IN SPIRITUAL EXPERIENCES

Let us now consider in detail some important aspects of spiritual experience, again using respondents' accounts to illustrate. First, what are the *qualities* that differentiate spiritual experiences from other experiences? Here are some examples, which by no means exhaust all the possibilities.

> *Deep inner silence, stillness, peace—pure being*
>
> I recently attended a workshop on walking the labyrinth. The leader had laid out a canvas replica of the labyrinth from Chartres cathedral. Grego-

rian chants were playing softly in the background. There was a faint smell of incense mixed with fresh flowers. As I began to walk the labyrinth, I was aware that I had to pay attention to the path painted on the canvas and that I was uncomfortable with the sharp turns, but soon I got used to it and just slowly walked. Then I sort of "zoned out" for a time and when I came out of it I was in the center of the labyrinth. I sat cross-legged on the floor for a long time and was filled with a comforting sense that I was "home."   *Woman, age 64*

Mental clarity: seeing, interpreting, and discerning meaning

In an airport bookstore in Anaheim, California, I picked up a little book called *The Impersonal Life*, a transcript of a divine message received by a man named Joseph Benner. I had never heard of him, but the book looked interesting. On the plane, I read: "Be *still*—and KNOW—I AM—GOD." I had read the words "Be still and know that I am God" many times in the Bible, but the cadence and emphasis here was different. It suggested that if I could be still within myself and focus on the "I Am" part of my experience, then I might directly experience God, and that would lead me to know God. That phrase has remained with me to this day. I have found it to be true, and trying to pay attention to the "I Am" is central to my spiritual life.   *Man, age 60*

Insight: sudden flashes of knowledge

In the fall of 1991 my grandmother died at age 88. About three months later, I had a dream that I was a little boy sitting on her lap. I was aware that I was no longer a little boy and that she was no longer living. As she stroked my shoulder, as she often did, she said, "There is love, there is forgiveness, and then there is peace." I woke up with a feeling that my grandmother had given me an incredible blessing. Those words have stuck with me, and I have made them into a personal mantra.   *Man, age 42*

Compassion: universal love in the face of suffering

My best friend was dying, and she was in a great deal of physical pain. I visited her each day, and to be present with her, instead of distancing myself from her pain by daydreaming, I had to muster all of the love I could find. Only limitless love allowed me to be present for that amount of pain. My friend and I met in that love each day.   *Man, age 52*

Connection with the ground of being[1]

I was driving down a country road on a sunny day, actually not thinking but just seeing the passing scenery. Gradually I became aware that the trees, the grass, the wildflowers, the sky, the road, and the car all began to shimmer with light. It was as if there was so much light within everything that it couldn't be contained, and the vividness of it was exhilarating. I realized that I, and everything around me, was completely permeated by God.

Man, age 67

Transcendence of personal self

I had inadvertently said something in a meeting that made my boss really mad. At the end of the meeting he said through clenched teeth, "I need to chat with you in my office *now!*" Unexpectedly, I felt a lack of fear. It was as if I was outside myself watching. In his office, he threw a major tantrum. I sat there calmly and quietly and did not respond in my usual defensive way. When he finally ran out of steam, I said, "I understand that you are angry about what happened, and I will not do that again." He said, "Well, OK." By my being able to stand outside my own feelings about what had happened, a situation that could have been ugly was neutralized.

Man, age 46

⌗

Nature is a fantastic teacher for me, and hiking is my religion. Leaving our fast-paced world behind, I walk in nature, overwhelmed by its majesty, and I just stop. Nature takes me outside myself and my personal concerns to focus on something much, much bigger and grander.

Man, age 58

Wonder

When I was eight, I spent the summer on a cousin's remote farm in the mountains of middle Tennessee. One of my chores was to shoo the cow and a couple of mules from the barnyard down a steep path to a spring about a quarter of a mile away. I did this twice each day. The morning run usually started at first light, just before sunrise. I would get up when I heard the birds, and by the time I dressed, ate a cold biscuit, and got to the barn there was plenty of light. Our little caravan usually moved pretty slowly over the side of the steep mountain and would get to the spring just about sunrise. I would sit on a stump while the animals drank and look at the sun coming through hundred-foot-high oak trees and be completely awestruck by the grandeur of nature.   *Man, age 72*

Inexpressibility

I look at my face in the mirror and see the ravages of time and gravity, the tracks of much laughter and some sadness, and the twinkle of the infinite in the eyes. I wink and smile.   *Man, age 73*

Mystery

When I first began to lose my hearing, I was frustrated that I could no longer effortlessly participate in things. I often didn't know what was going on because I couldn't hear the discussion or directions or whatever. I tried reading lips but never really got the hang of it. Then I began trying to simply "be" with the people—to merely be there with them, to look gently into their eyes, to sense their energy. It was an amazingly pleasant experience, and I would often smile a little, which seemed to make people relax. My world is mostly silent now, and I have lots of friends to guide me through it safely.   *Man, age 85*

Paradox

When I finally let go of my strong attachment to growing spiritually, I grew much faster than I had before.   *Woman, age 48*

Immateriality and intangibility

I was hiking alone in the mountains, going up a winding trail that steadily rose up the north side of a steep wooded slope. I came to a switchback in the trail that crossed a rocky creek bed. The creek was running full and I stooped to feel the ice-cold water from the spring melting of the snow pack. I sat on a large rock and listened to the soothing sound of the rushing water, the chirping of birds, and the wind in the trees. The creek banks were teeming with mosses and wildflowers of many colors. I sat there for several minutes taking it all in. Then it dawned on me, "This is a holy place." It was holy because it drew from me feelings of deep tenderness, awe, and warm appreciation. I sat there for twenty minutes or so, then with a feeling of deep fulfillment, I happily walked back the way I had come.   *Woman, age 68*

Motivation to focus on one's spiritual journey

A few years ago I attended a meditation retreat in Indianapolis. After some brief instructions, we spent three hours sitting on the floor, each of us silently repeating a personal mantra. During this time, I struggled to concentrate, and when my mind would wander, it was an effort to gently bring my attention back to the mantra. The morning session was followed by about twenty minutes of chanting. The afternoon meditation session was to be another three hours. About a half-hour into the afternoon session, I felt my awareness leaving the mantra, but the mind was nowhere to be seen. I was awake and alert but there were no body sensations or thoughts. This was a blissful experience, relaxed and peaceful. I remained in this state for most of the afternoon session. I have experienced this many times since, but that was my first time.   *Woman, age 52*

Transformation

After I finished my first yoga class, I got into my car and had a strong impression that something big was happening to me. The rest of that day I was aware of what was happening in each moment in a way that I had never been before. I was intensely aware—of the scents in the building, the skin of my fingers on my computer keyboard, the amazing sound of my breathing. It was incredible to recognize and be present to everything that was happening and most of all to realize that everything had an impact on me.   *Woman, age 36*

To be defined as spiritual, experiences do not necessarily have to have all of the qualities illustrated above. Some spiritual experiences consist mainly of wonder and feelings of connection, others are primarily experiences of compassion, and others are mainly of silence, space, and intangibility.

AVENUES OF SPIRITUAL EXPERIENCE

So where do we look in our being for these qualities? There are many avenues or channels through which we receive spiritual experiences. Here are some avenues and typical spiritual experiences we might have through those avenues, again illustrated by examples from my respondents.

Physical: deep peace, quietude, and stillness; goose bumps

When I was nine, I usually went to church alone. My mother's only day off work was Sunday, and my grandmother was in ill health. I would get to church an hour or more before anything started so that I could be alone in the big sanctuary, with its smells of old hymnals, candles, and wood polish. The early-morning sun through the stained-glass windows cast beautiful patterns on the walls, and there was real stillness there.

Man, age 69

Sensory: esthetic wonder (art, music, nature)

A friend of mine died, and I attended his funeral, which was held in a Methodist church. I had attended church regularly as a teenager and had sung in the church choir, so I knew many hymns. As we rose and began to sing a familiar hymn, I became so choked up I could barely continue to sing. I felt a great opening of spirit. I don't think it was the words of the hymn that brought on this experience so much as the resonance and harmony of all the voices that drew me to a sacred space within myself.

Woman, age 64

I was playing my guitar, trying out a new chord progression, when the sound and rhythm clicked my mind into a new gear and my awareness into another type of consciousness in which I was just playing and was with that song and only that song.   *Man, age 32*

*Consciousness/Awareness: intense presence and
transcendent spaciousness*

The degree to which I am present, whether it is in gardening, giving a hug, dancing, communing with nature, or making love, determines whether the experience is "spiritual" or not. All experiences are spiritual if that is one's orientation!   *Woman, age 47*

The summer after first grade, I attended a vacation Bible school, and at the conclusion of the week the kids put on a program for parents. I was an enthusiastic singer (read loud), and I was given a solo to sing, *This Little Light of Mine*. As I sang I realized that I was singing about something that was *actually within me*. I could feel it. Seventy years later, that feeling is still there.   *Man, age 76*

Thought: integrative, holistic [2]

When I was a boy, I attended a boarding school where we spent great energy memorizing psalms. Now I am old, hard of hearing, and blind, and I find great pleasure in being able to recall these psalms from my memory. I sometimes feel moved to recite a psalm for friends, and I am so at home with the text that I feel I can go beyond the text to touch the source from which the psalm came.   *Man, age 89*

Relational: social access to feelings of spiritual connection

My mother and I had had an uneasy relationship for most of my life. On the one hand, I felt much loved by her, but on the other hand, no one, including me, ever eluded her critical eye. One day we were having one of our "knock-down, drag-out" exchanges when suddenly we stopped talking, looked at each other for a long moment, and simultaneously broke into raucous laughter. We realized how wonderfully connected we were at a deep, deep level that was completely untouched by the melodrama we created. Our disagreements were never the same after that. They had a new underlying gentleness and much less edge.   *Man, age 40*

⊕

A few weeks ago, I was contemplating the energy of all the generations of mothers in my family that had gone before me, from my great-grandmother to my grandmothers, to my mother. In the midst of this I got a clear message from my mother, who died ten years ago. We'd never had a good relationship, and there was no great emotional tie—at least, I didn't think so, but I got the message from her, "Everything I did was out of love for you. I was afraid for you." I knew then that she loved me and that love is stronger than death.   *Woman, age 67*

Intuitive/Mystical: contemplative knowing, waiting

Today is my birthday. Last night I started thinking about my life so far. I realized that I have been consciously present for twenty-seven years. One day I will not have this body. I knew this, but right now I feel it. My daughter will most likely outlive me. There will be a time when I am not here with her. I do believe that I will "be" even after death, but not like this. It's amazing to feel and share this. I will not always be me in this shape.   *Woman, age 27*

Unitive: complete transcendence—absence of "other"

There are times when I look into the eyes of my 2-year-old granddaughter and am instantly transported into a feeling of being part of everything, as if all the mysteries of the universe and my place in it are of no consequence at all.   *Man, age 57*

Thus, there are many avenues through which we may experience the spiritual qualities of life. As we look at the qualities and avenues of spiritual experience depicted in tables 3 and 4, we can see that spiritual experience is enormously multifaceted.

The word *spiritual* can also be used as an adjective to modify a large number of aspects of life. Table 5 lists some examples with brief definitions. These terms and definitions sketch out conceptual, linguistic territory relating to the spiritual region of life and can be used to have conversations, share experiences, and conduct research on spirituality as a topic in its own right. If we want to know the extent to which spiritual concerns permeate a person's life, we need to ask about many of the items on this list, which does not provide answers so much as give us a way to identify and frame questions. Certainly all these aspects of spirituality are salient for understanding the relation between spirituality and aging.

Given the robust public interest in spirituality, the conceptual narrowness of current discussions about spirituality and aging within the field of aging itself is difficult to understand. Certainly spirituality is a central source of life satisfaction for a large proportion of aging and older people. Why have gerontologists lagged so far behind the public in developing a language of spirituality?

TABLE 3
Qualities of Spiritual Experience

Pure being: deep inner space, silence, stillness, peace, equanimity
Discernment: clarity of seeing, interpreting, and meaning
Compassion: universal love in the face of suffering
Connection with the ground of being, direct and conscious
Transcending the personal self, "witness" consciousness
Wonder and inexpressibility, comfort with mystery and paradox
Immateriality and intangibility
Confidence and trust in spiritual process
Earnestness and motivation for a spiritual journey
Transformation

TABLE 4
Avenues and Types of Spiritual Experience

Physical: deep peace, quietude, and stillness
Sensory: esthetic wonder
Consciousness/Awareness: many levels and stages
Thought
Intuitive/Mystical: contemplative knowing, waiting
Unitive: complete transcendence, absence of "other"

First, the conflation of religion and spirituality has inhibited scholars from pursuing the emerging interest in spirituality as a topic of its own. Our scientific world has been so bent on protecting itself from religion that it has created blinders that prevent us from understanding spirituality. We do not have to become a rock to study rocks, but we do have to understand the nature of "rockness." Likewise, to understand spirituality we have to at least make an attempt to understand how those who have come into direct contact with the essence of spirituality experience their inner world.

Second, gerontologists tend to be uninformed about the existing literature on spirituality. Much of this literature was written many years ago and tends not to show up in literature searches that are limited to academic articles published over the past ten years. To begin to understand the complex nature of the inner spiritual life, we do not have to begin from scratch. There are useful anthologies that bring together wisdom from the sages of many spiritual traditions (Hixon 1978; Huxley 1944; James 1905 [2005]; Mitchell 1989, 1991; Vardey 1995). These texts help us understand various concepts surrounding spirituality by triangulation. Spirituality is by definition a sensitizing concept that refers to a conceptual and experiential inner region. To get at the essence of such concepts, it helps to have access to several statements from different scholars. As we read many expressions of the same issue, we are more likely to find the essence of the issue. This process is essential background for studying spirituality and aging, and the anthologies listed above are a good place to start.

CONCLUSION

Spirituality is a broad term rooted in inner experience. A large majority of adults report having experiences they deem spiritual. Spiritual experiences are interpreted through three types of consciousness: intense awareness of

TABLE 5
Aspects of Spiritual Experience

Spiritual experience: spiritual qualities and avenues directly observed and lived through

Spiritual states: ways or forms of being that reflect spiritual qualities and may occur through various spiritual avenues. Sometimes spiritual states appear to progress through stages or levels

Spiritual capacity: the potentiality, capability, or practical ability to be aware of spiritual qualities and avenues

Spiritual history: spiritual experiences and learning that are consciously or nonconsciously remembered, interpreted, and integrated into a personal spiritual narrative

Spiritual concepts and language: ideas and language used to describe, interpret, and motivate spiritual experience

Spiritual connection: a subjective perception of physical, mental, and mystical connection with the ground of being arising through various avenues of spiritual experience

Spiritual practice: actions intended to acknowledge, celebrate, or encourage the experience of spiritual qualities and avenues. Examples include meditation, prayer, contemplation, and habits such as mindfulness, waiting, and letting go

Spiritual knowledge: a person's experience-based spiritual awareness and understanding, including integrated memories, comprehension, discernment, and clear grasp of spiritual meaning

Spiritual process: a person's way of observing, interpreting, and integrating experiences of spiritual qualities and avenues, learned through life experience

Spiritual persistence: the extent to which a person is repeatedly motivated and drawn to focus attention on spiritual avenues and qualities

Spiritual mystery: the ineffable nature of the ground of being and the pure beingness within our experience

Spiritual piety: spiritual experience related to religion; devotion, righteousness, or otherworldliness

Spiritual being: an experience of pure presence, both immanent and transcendent

Spiritual energy: physical and psychic energy arising from the experience of spiritual qualities

Spiritual growth: developing or evolving greater spiritual capacity or a more effective spiritual process

Spiritual breakthrough: pushing through a spiritual difficulty or obstacle, thereby making further spiritual progress possible

Spiritual transmission: sending spiritual knowledge, practice, or understanding from one person to another

Spiritual transformation: a marked change that transcends a previous form of spiritual capacity or integration, at times leading to or following from religious conversion

Spiritual community: a group centered on spiritual pursuits and spiritual being, within which members can meet many of their needs for meaning, belonging, constructive feedback, aid, comfort, guidance, and opportunities to serve

---

the present; "witness" consciousness, which transcends the personal self; and transcendent awareness, which is open to the presence of the sacred. For many people, these types of consciousness, although distinctive, can reside in a person's being simultaneously.

In this chapter, spiritual experiences were described by many individuals, each in his or her unique language and conceptual framework. Spiritual experience can be found in many different contexts, including life experiences wherever they happen, religious services and environments, nature, relating with others, community service, and work. Qualities that characterize spiritual experiences include inner stillness, mental clarity, insight, compassion, connection with the ground of being, wonder, inexpressibility, mystery, paradox, personal transformation, and motivation to continue a spiritual journey. Spiritual experiences come through a variety of channels or avenues within consciousness: physical or sensory events, nonverbal awareness, verbal thought, relational awareness, mystical states, or unitive states, in which the individual merges for a time with the ground of being. When people use *spiritual* as an adjective to modify various aspects of life, such as personal history or aspirations, they may become aware of many venues in which to look for experiences that could be called spiritual or spiritually conditioned.

At this point, it should be obvious that the nature of spiritual experience is complex and does not lend itself to simplistic concepts or measures. Now I will add even more complexity by putting all this in motion in a discussion of spiritual development.

✤ ✤ ✤ ✤

Spiritual Development

The previous chapter described a spiritual region of human experience characterized by identifiable qualities, occurring through several avenues of experience and accompanying many aspects of life. Awareness of this region and experience with it vary greatly among people and also evolve over time for most. Questions that guide this chapter include: What does it mean to grow spiritually? Is spiritual development influenced by personal spiritual aspirations? Does spiritual evolution occur in stages or is it continuous or is it both? Does the capacity for spiritual experience evolve?

Just as we can study a person's physical, psychological, or social development, we can also study her or his spiritual development. And just as physical, psychological, and social development are complex topics, so is spiritual development. We begin this chapter with a brief discussion of various ways to conceptualize that development. We then consider how these various conceptions play out when applied to spiritual development.

BACKGROUND

Historically, ideas about development have been rooted in the physical life cycle of living organisms. Plants and animals have genetically programmed life spans in which they grow to maturity, enjoy some period of full maturity, and then begin to decline physically and eventually die. This is called the maturation-maturity-aging model. Does development occur during all three stages or just during the stage leading up to full maturity? Early conceptions of development held that once child and adolescent development were completed, development was over, and life was simply a playing out of early destiny. There was little conception that development could continue into later adulthood.

In the 1970s, research on middle-aged and older adults began to show that previously unused physical and mental capabilities could be awakened and developed in adults of any age (Riley and Foner 1968), that numerous psychological traits continued to evolve and improve well into old age (Salthouse 1982), and that social environments made a big difference by demanding, encouraging, or discouraging continued development in midlife and later (Cohen 2000). Scholars began to look not just at deficits of aging but also at undeveloped potentials for development in later life.

Interestingly, recorded history contains many illustrations of middle-aged and older adults having the capacity to continue to develop spiritually. Late-life spiritual development is present in historical records from a wide variety of cultures and historical eras. However, this information came from the humanities—history, anthropology, religious studies, and philosophy—and was largely ignored by scholars in the social sciences as they developed social gerontology.

In the early days of the twentieth century, most people thought spiritual development was the province of religion, not science. For example, William James's (1905[2005]) classic treatise on subjective spirituality was titled *The Varieties of Religious Experience. Spirituality* was not a word in common use then. The beginnings of gerontology were mostly silent on the subject. For example, there was no material on spirituality in the *Handbook of Social Gerontology* (Tibbitts 1960), only a chapter on organized religion, and the *Handbook of Aging and the Individual* (Birren 1959), which dealt with psychology, contained no mention of either spirituality or religion.

By the 1950s, much of science was antagonistic toward subjective inner development, stressing conformity instead. A "secular humanist" view supported an image of principled science that did not depend on religion, which was seen as opposed to the flexibility of thought needed for science. Religions' theological definitions of reality were seen as conflicting with empiricism. The doctrine of separation of church and state was used to justify exclusion of religion from publicly funded education and research. Spirituality was seen in that era as an offshoot of religion, which caused spirituality also to be disvalued as a subject of study.

The "human potential movement" of the 1960s challenged this view by claiming that human beings had many untapped capabilities and that taking responsibility for our own development was the key to discovering and developing our potentials. This movement gave rise to an enormous "self-help" culture, which encouraged adults to exert influence on their own development. Spirituality was a major area of untapped potential identified by workers in the self-help field. Unfortunately, scientific research has contributed little to the conversation about what spiritual development is and how it can be nurtured or hindered.

Despite a negative climate for the study of spirituality and spiritual development, several developmental perspectives were created that can serve as orienting frameworks for inquiry about spiritual development and how it relates to aging. Some are offshoots of general theories of human development; others were created primarily to explain development in later adulthood.

ERIK H. ERIKSON

In 1955, psychologist Erik Erikson published *Childhood and Society*, which was mainly about child development but also contained brief discussions of developmental issues of young adulthood, middle adulthood, and old age. Erikson's ideas on this subject evolved considerably over the years, with major revisions to his "life stages of psychosocial development" published in 1963, 1986, and 1997. Erikson's theory has had considerable influence as an overview, and the later revisions of the theory reflect an increasing emphasis on spirituality as a developmental theme in the later stages of life.

In Erikson's framework, development focused on doing what was psychologically needed to arrive at an identity of oneself as loving, competent, and good in the social context of successive age-appropriate life stages. Movement from one life stage to another was contingent on resolving the "psychosocial crisis" inherent in a given life stage in order to move on to the next. Each succeeding life stage often also involved review and reconsideration of the resolutions of earlier life stages. This was especially likely in the old age life stage (Erikson, Erikson, and Kivnick 1986).

Table 6 shows the 1986 version of Erikson's life stages, with the main developmental issue and typical resolution for each stage. Note that Erikson never attached chronological age definitions to these life stages. At the heart of this formulation is the idea that as we grow, achieve maturity, and age, we are confronted with a predictable set of dilemmas associated with each life stage. These dilemmas arise from having to adapt inwardly to changes that come with moving from one culturally defined life stage to another. Resolving these dilemmas does not involve choosing one side of the dilemma and

TABLE 6
Erikson's Life Stage Theory of Psychosocial Development

Life Stage	Psychosocial Tension	Balancing Resolution
Old age	Integrity versus despair	Wisdom
Adulthood	Generativity versus self-absorption	Care
Young adulthood	Intimacy versus isolation	Love
Adolescence	Identity versus confusion	Fidelity (to worldview)
School age	Industry versus inferiority	Competence
Play age	Initiative versus guilt	Purpose
Early childhood	Autonomy versus shame and doubt	Will
Infancy	Basic trust versus basic mistrust	Hope

Source: Adapted from Erikson, Erikson, and Kivnick (1986, 36).

expunging the other. "Successful" resolution involves creating a balance that acknowledges the reality of both sides of the dilemma. So, for example, in infancy "trust is mandatory: but . . . it can exist positively only in juxtaposition with a 'sensible' mistrust—also necessary for existence" (ibid., 38). Each developmental dilemma involves creating ways that we can acknowledge and accept both positive and negative experiences of ourselves.

Spirituality finds its way into Erikson's framework through the gradual emergence of a type of consciousness that Erikson says comes increasingly into play in "vital involvement," which results in a "heightened awareness that can by no means necessarily be claimed by the usual 'ego'" (ibid., 51). Erikson defined this consciousness as a special kind of "I," a basic awareness of existence. This is the "I am" of which I wrote earlier.

Using Erikson's framework, we can see the young adult's quest for intimacy, the adult's concern for generativity, and the older person's transcendent wisdom as involving successive increases in capacity to stand outside one's own self-centered agendas and feel connection and concern for things larger than oneself. This capacity is rooted in existential spirituality. The "sense of 'I,' in old age, still has a once-for-all chance of transcending time-bound identities and sensing, if only in the simplest terms, an all-human and existential identity which world religions have attempted to create" (ibid., 53).

The developmental issue of young adulthood, according the Erikson, is intimacy versus isolation. To avoid a life of isolation, adults must develop the capacity for eventual commitment to lasting friendships, companionship, and sexual mutuality. This requires the capacity to stand outside ourselves and empathize with another.

In midlife, the issue is generativity versus self-absorption. Generativity is taking care of what has been and is being "procreated, produced, and created." To develop this capacity, we must be able to see our needs in a context that includes the needs of others and be able to put others' needs ahead of ours when appropriate. Thus, generativity extends the circle of empathy developed in young adulthood to adjacent generations in the family, at work, and in the community. At the center of this capacity is a growing strength of nonpersonal consciousness.

In old age, the issue is integrity versus despair. Integrity is being able to stand back from the mosaic of one's multitude of characteristics and life experiences, both positive and negative, and see this mosaic as an interconnected whole. To do this, we have to be able to look directly at our negative qualities and life experiences, accept them, and move on into being who we are. If we can't do this, then negative personal qualities and experiences can drag us into despair. Having practice focusing on the "I am" of pure being gives us a place to reside in our awareness where we can look at all aspects of ourselves with compassion. It is a place from which we can forgive our past and clearly see hope in the way forward. Integrity is not denial; it is acceptance and compassion for the being that is.

LARS TORNSTAM

In *The Life Cycle Completed*, published following Erik Erikson's death, Joan Erikson (1997) cited Lars Tornstam's theory of gerotranscendence as a ninth stage of development that could also occur in old age. Gerotranscendence theory asserts that spiritual development gradually and steadily increases from middle age onward and results in a shift from a materialistic, role-oriented life philosophy to a transcendent, spiritual perspective in late old age (Tornstam 2005). Gerotranscendence is present to some extent in most aging adults, according to the theory, but becomes a prevalent metaperspective mainly in adults over 70. Gerotranscendence theory presumes that spiritual development is intrinsic, but the exact source of this development is unspecified. Nevertheless, this development can be promoted or stifled by social factors such as language and normative constraints, opportunity structures, social class, and education. Thus, the degree of gerotranscendence varies even within the very old population.

The broadened spiritual perspective that typifies mature gerotranscendence is indicated by three dimensions. In the cosmic dimension, concepts such as life, death, space, and time are seen as involving an element of mystery and are seen against a backdrop of infinity. In the self-transcendent dimension, the personal self is no longer the center of attention, and there is increased honesty and acceptance about the personal self. In the social selectivity dimension, relationships focus mainly on close friends and family, and much less energy is spent relating to casual acquaintances and strangers, with a consequent increase in solitude and less emphasis on pro forma role playing. Attitudes toward material possessions shift from acquisition to maintaining the bare essentials for a comfortable life. Social selectivity leads to a much more thoughtful, contemplative stance toward relationships, activities, and lifestyles. Gerotranscendence results in less concern with social conformity for conformity's sake. Mature gerotranscendence may make for a different type of effective participation in the community rather than for disengagement.

Historically, the role of elder in the community was assumed to have a spiritual element. Elders were seen not only as keepers of spiritual traditions but also as human beings who had benefited from decades of spiritual development. While most communities no longer assume that spiritual development is connected with lengthy life experience and do not ascribe the role of elder to all older people, there are important vestiges of the functional role of spiritual elders, especially in families but also in friendship networks and in spiritual communities.

Sages are people who can manifest wisdom and retain a strong spiritual connection in the face of life's trials. Most sages are old people. In the stages and processes through which aging people develop into sages we get a glimmer of the internal processes that complement the theory of gerotranscendence (Atchley 2003).

Erikson's and Tornstam's perspectives on spiritual development both echo the ancient Hindu Vedas, dating back at least four thousand years, which describe various stages of spiritual development tied to stages of life. The Vedas state that when a householder experiences the birth of the first grandchild, it is time to begin a process of turning away from material and political concerns and toward spiritual concerns. Note that the triggering event for beginning this shift is familial, not chronological. In the era in which the Vedas were written, grandparenthood often first occurred when parents were in their late 30s or early 40s. Thus, the idea of people turning to spiritual concerns in midlife and later has been around a long time.

The link with grandparenthood is interesting. Many grandparents experience grandparenthood as a shift away from the responsibility and accountability associated with child rearing toward a purely generative relationship with their grandchildren. For many grandparents, the role emphasizes an existential quality of relationship rather than a functional quality of mere caretaking.

In present-day society, retirement may represent a similar opportunity to turn toward spiritual concerns. Indeed, retirees form a sizable share of the market for workshops and retreats that focus on spiritual growth and development.

HARRY R. MOODY AND DAVID A. CARROLL

In *The Five Stages of the Soul*, Harry R. "Rick" Moody and David Carroll (1997) present a different kind of stage theory of spiritual development. Erikson's theory of spiritual development is driven primarily by an "outside-in" process of adapting to stimuli from the external demands of integrating oneself with a sociocultural life course. Moody and Carroll's theory takes a deeper, "inside-out" approach, in which development is driven not so much by external processes as by internal ones. Although hypothetically a person could begin this process at any age, most of the life histories the authors cite were from middle-aged and older adults. Moody and Carroll envision spiritual development as a continuous series of small, often gradual and subtle changes that take place in the context of a profound shift in perspective, involving a strong sense of spiritual connection and enlightenment. At the heart of the theory is the assumption that the soul—human spiritual capacity—is real and in most people has been covered over by language and social conditioning. The stages of the soul are about a process of reconnecting with one's spiritual nature and integrating that spiritual nature into one's physical, psychological, and social nature.

Moody and Carroll's stages of the soul—the shift from an unconscious spiritual life to a conscious spiritual life—are as follows:

— *The Call:* The person has experiences that indicate a deeper aspect of human existence than previously known. He or she feels drawn to explore this "hidden-in-plain-sight" field of possibility and is attracted, led, or drawn back to this aspect over and over again.
— *The Search:* The person searches inwardly for signs of spiritual experience and also searches for teachers, texts, experiences, and practices that can help her or him glimpse spiritual nature. There is a thirst for dwelling in this particular mystery.

— *The Struggle:* The person struggles with letting go of old ways of seeing and behaving, facing doubts and fears of failure, and developing routine practices that create openings for experiences of spiritual connection and transcendence. Spiritual community is often a particularly important support during this stage.

— *The Breakthrough:* The person emerges from the struggle into stunning clarity of spiritual perception and purpose. The person breaks through into new qualities of experience: timelessness and immense space, more accurate perception of "reality," "lightness of being"—liberation, deep inner silence, stillness and peace, loss of fears about death, a sense of new beginning, feelings of universal love and compassion, and a profound sense that what has happened cannot be captured in words.

— *The Return:* The person who experiences a breakthrough then experiences that life goes on. The new way of being needs to be integrated into daily life, and the person feels a responsibility to give back in return for the amazing gift received. There is no standard form to the return; returns are shaped by personality, circumstances, and culture. Many if not most returns are invisible except to the persons experiencing them.

In *The Five Stages of the Soul*, this framework is fleshed out with dozens of examples taken from Moody's interviews.[1] This approach allows us to hear these abstract stages expressed in the words of people going through them.

Moody and Carroll's framework is an extraordinary resource for researchers and practitioners who wish to include spirituality as a topic in research and practice. It is also well received by students and general readers interested in a spiritual journey. However, Ruth Ray and Susan McFadden (2001) criticized this framework as being too linear, too stylized, and a recreation of Joseph Campbell's *Hero with a Thousand Faces* (1972). Ray and McFadden's alternative perspective on spiritual development is discussed later in this chapter.

Moody used a feedback-systems approach in developing the conceptual framework. He drew ideas skillfully from a broad sweep of writings on spirituality in philosophy, literature, poetry, and religion from many times and places. Then he used his tentative framework to structure in-depth interviews with more than a hundred knowledgeable informants, people with experience of the spiritual journey. He allowed his ideas to be shaped and disciplined by his respondents. He also took the ideas out into the community in the form of workshops. The feedback from participants refined his ideas. Moody himself has been on a conscious spiritual journey for many years, and that experience gave him an important ability to see patterns within what he was reading and hearing from respondents. Moody's experience illustrates well the power of combining interpretive and storytelling methods from the humanities with data-gathering approaches common in the social sciences. The result is richer and deeper than the usual scholarly study.

I use a framework similar to Moody's to describe more modest, ongoing cycles of spiritual development. To avoid confusion of terminology, I use different labels for phases of short-term spiritual development. Table 7 shows a comparison of Moody's big-picture labels with the labels I use for shorter cycles of spiritual development.

— *Awakening Interest:* Something happens to heighten awareness of the possibility of further spiritual growth. Many people on a spiritual journey read and attend study groups, discussion groups, and educational programs at least partly to heighten their chance of discovering new spiritual possibilities.
— *Inquiry:* Following curiosity about a possibility by pursuing study, discussion, reflection, or contemplation and being open to discovery.
— *Endeavor:* Developing new practices, creating new routines, being patient and waiting in the face of frustration. Dealing with discomfort, confusion, uncertainty, loss of inspiration, ambivalence, or disheartenment.
— *Integration:* New pieces combine with old pieces to form a new big picture.
— *Intention:* Forming a new or renewed sense of spiritual direction.

TABLE 7
Phases in a Cycle of Spiritual Development

Phase Label		
Moody and Carroll	Atchley	What Happens
Call	Awakening interest	Opening, attraction, something missing, yearning
Search	Inquiry	Study, discussion, contemplation, scanning
Struggle	Endeavor	Establishing practices; creating a groove; dealing with discomfort, confusion, uncertainty, loss of inspiration, ambivalence, or disheartenment
Breakthrough	Integration	Pieces fall together to form a big picture
Return	Intention	Newly developed or renewed sense of spiritual direction

Source: Adapted from Moody and Carroll (1997); labels for short-term development by the author.

For many people, this process is experienced as an upward spiral of increasing scope and clarity. Even while a person may be in one of Moody and Carroll's stages of the soul, such as struggle, there may be within that stage several cycles of increasing understanding before the person experiences a breakthrough. However, this idea of upward spiral is just a description of what seems to happen; it should not be taken as deterministic or inevitable.

KEN WILBER

In *Integral Spirituality* (Wilber 2006), Ken Wilber summarizes more than twenty years' work in organizing and presenting his thoughts on spiritual development. The major strength of this work is its panoramic scope, including perspectives from a wide variety of bodies of thought. Wilber is a master at providing diagrams that help the reader visualize relationships and patterns within a large number of abstract concepts. Here are some quotes that give a hint of the richness of Wilber's work as a source of concepts and hypotheses about spiritual development:

> Your consciousness is struggling to move not only horizontally through [various] states but vertically through stages. (2006, 138)

>   ⁂

> [Verticality] is consciousness per se. Thus, "degree of consciousness" is itself altitude: the more consciousness, the higher the altitude (subconscious to self-conscious to superconscious). In this view, all the developmental lines move through the same altitude gradient. (2006, 65)

>   ⁂

> There is not one line of development that the dozens of [developmental theories] are giving different maps of; rather, there are at least a dozen different developmental lines—cognitive, moral, interpersonal, emotional, psychosexual, kinesthetic, self, values, needs, and so on. (2002, 58)

>   ⁂

> All of [these] lines can then be aligned . . . , moving through the same altitude gradient (as well as moving through their own specific structures or stages). (2006, 65)

>   ⁂

> Sometimes people speak of something like "spiritual intelligence," which not only is available at the highest levels in any of the [developmental] lines, but is *its own developmental line.* . . . "Spiritual" is not something that refers

only to the highest, transpersonal, and transrational levels in various developmental lines, but is something that has its own first, second, and third tiers (or structure-stages). (2006, 101)

Integral Spirituality packs 300 pages with dense, abstract, conceptual prose that requires of the reader a considerable background in psychology, sociology, philosophy, comparative religion, and many other subjects. Nevertheless, it is a treasure trove of ideas about spirituality and spiritual development. From our point of view, a major weakness of the work is that Wilber does not see aging or life stages as important factors in the process of spiritual development. It would take a major endeavor to integrate Wilber's perspective with our knowledge base about how physical, psychological, and social aging interacts with human development.

JAMES FOWLER

Fowler (1981) described stages of faith development. He defined faith as "the dynamic patterns by which we find life's meaning." Fowler's (1981, 1991) theory conceives of faith development in adulthood as having three stages: individuative-reflective faith, which could begin in the early twenties, in which the self begins to turn away from external sources of spiritual authority toward the development of an internal moral and spiritual orientation that has meaning for the individual; conjunctive faith, beginning in midlife or later and involving acceptance of paradox and ambiguity, a deepening sense of understanding, disillusionment with the over-reliance on logic and rational thought that is typical in the individuative-reflective stage, and a more open attitude toward religious traditions other than one's own; and finally, universalizing faith, occurring late in life and involving a rare willingness to give up one's life to make values a reality on earth. Fowler's exemplars of people who achieved the last stage include Mahatma Gandhi, Thomas Merton, and Mother Teresa. Fowler felt that most adults probably never progress beyond the individuative-reflective faith, even in very old age. Fowler's theory has been criticized for relying too much on cognitive concepts of spirituality (Koenig 1995a).

RUTH RAY AND SUSAN MCFADDEN

Ruth Ray and Susan McFadden (2001) offer two metaphors—the web and the quilt—as alternatives to the "hero's journey" metaphor of spiritual development offered by Moody and Carroll (1997). They begin with a critique based on the limitations of stage models in capturing the meandering quality of many spiritual journeys. In particular, they criticize Moody and Carroll for over-reaching assertions, such as "a clear pattern of spiritual stages does exist" and it "runs deep in our blood" (9). Ray and McFadden also point out that many accounts of spiritual development, particularly those of women and minorities, do not interpret spiritual growth in terms of the "solo quest narrative" (202). They emphasize the interpersonal context in which many if not most spiritual journeys occur. A big part of the creation of personal meaning, including spiritual meaning, occurs in the exchange of ideas with other people. (Kahn and Antonucci [1981] referred to this as the "convoy of social support," another metaphor I like.)

As metaphor, the web concept implies a loosely woven yet strong structure. Part of a web can be destroyed without compromising the functioning of the overall structure. A web has a large number of interconnections. The network concept is a similar idea. The Internet is a vast network, a sea of relational possibilities that is enormously flexible in its capacity to respond to individual needs. Personal networks are also effective in supporting both the development and the maintenance of networks and meeting the needs of their individual members. Spiritual webs or networks are a group context within which individuals can develop spiritual capacity and spiritual identity. I have no doubt that networks of spiritual friends and spiritual teachers are hugely important influences on the spiritual journeys of most people, but this will remain a hypothesis until it is studied. Exactly how webs support the spiritual journey remains to be discovered.

> A *quilt* has multiple layers and is crafted over time. Like the individual differences found in ways of being spiritual, some people's quilts have an organizing structure immediately apparent to all; others' are of the "crazy-quilt" variety that, when viewed partially may make little sense, but can be quite beautiful when seen as a whole. Quilts, like spirituality, may have different functions at different points in the life span. . . A very important aspect of quilt making is that although parts of the quilt (its "blocks") may be crafted individually, the whole quilt is traditionally the outcome of people gathering to stitch it together. . . As spirituality is nurtured across the life span through relationships with others, the 'stitches' of those relational encounters may be quite hard to distinguish when viewed in the context of the whole pattern of life. Nevertheless, without them, there could be no holistic, integrated sense of spirituality. (Ray and McFadden 2001, 205).

This perspective argues strongly for balancing individualism with relational aspects as we attempt to understand spiritual development.

Ray and McFadden cite an example of three women who went on a spiritual retreat together—just the three of them. "We had grown stronger spiritually. We knew we were three small miracles in the universe, three women trying to fit into Nature, three women feeling connected to all people because all of us are born in the same womb. Each of us, to herself, made a promise to grow stronger still in the months and years ahead by seeking spiritually and expressing spirituality in relationships with others" (Wade-Gayles and Finch 1995, 84). In this context of mutual support, these women had made commitments to their future spiritual development.

SPIRITUAL DEVELOPMENT AND THE LOSS OF COGNITIVE ABILITY

It is true that being able to conceptualize and recall one's spiritual journey depends on retaining the ability to use language and to access one's spiritual experiences, ideas, and history from memory. But what happens for those who experience dementia? Does dementia mean the gradual loss of personhood, including spiritual capacity and identity? There has been little research on this subject, but I can sketch out some ideas that might serve as useful orientation on this question. Short-term memory is usually one of the first functions affected by dementia. People who experience memory impairment may not be able to remember well what happened to them yesterday, so their recent recall of spiritual experiences may be limited, but their ability to recall various elements of their spiritual history throughout adulthood may remain remarkably intact. Mrs. E is a good example:

> Mrs. E cannot tell you what she had for lunch or what activities she engaged in yesterday, and she cannot remember the names of any of her caregivers in the nursing home. But she can remember in vivid detail the church services she attended with her children when they were "little," the words of hymns they sang, and aspects of the church building she found beautiful. She recalls that the church was just across the street from her grandmother's house. More than that, she can tell you what she learned in that church and how her life experiences dovetailed with the Christian social teachings of the "Golden Rule," kindness toward strangers and the poor, the importance of peace among men, and leading an

upright life. She recalls many stories from her family history that clearly illustrate the morals of various Bible stories through both positive and negative examples. Even though she cannot track her current life experiences well, she still has a strong sense of personal spiritual identity and spiritually based morality. Her gregarious personality is still very much intact.

People in more advanced stages of dementia may lose much of their ability to recall even distant memories, yet in most cases they still have a strong connection with the present. Many people with advanced dementia may not be able to tell you much about who or where they are or who the people around them are, but they still exhibit many of the traits we prize most in personhood—kindness toward others, listening to the life stories of others, and caring for one another. Frances Hellebrandt (1978) presented an early useful portrait of this aspect of dementia. Based on long-term observations of residents of a locked dementia ward, Hellebrandt, herself 76, described the daily existence of sixteen residents.

> They move about freely, often in pairs, showing evidence of concern for one another even though they never address each other by name and cannot identify the person with whom they are walking. . . . They are clean, neat, and groomed appropriately, for the most part. On occasion they may wear two or three dresses at once. . . . The casual observer would find the group deceptively normal.
>
> All residents in the locked ward are completely disoriented as to place, time, day, date, year, seasons, or holidays. They have a poor memory for ongoing events. . . None knows that their behavior is in any way aberrant. Neither do they realize they live in an institution. Yet much of what we consider positive human qualities remain alive in these people—concern for others, friendliness, and optimism (68).

We could make the argument, based on our definition of basic spirituality as *beingness*, that as long as there is being there is the possibility of spirituality, and as long as there is spirituality, there is a right to be considered a person. In fact, the experience of beingness may be the last experience to be lost to dementia.

THE SOCIAL CONTEXT OF SPIRITUAL DEVELOPMENT

Spiritual development can occur spontaneously and without group support. However, most people use group connections with friends, coworkers, family members, or members of their spiritual or religious community to support them at each stage or throughout the process of spiritual evolution.

Buddhists speak of the "three jewels" of Buddhism: the Buddha, the Dharma, and the Sangha. The Buddha symbolizes the possibility of enlightenment in this lifetime. The Dharma refers to a principled way of life that is continuously revealed to those who lead a contemplative life. The Sangha is the contemplative spiritual community that can serve as protection for each member against the possibility that spiritual realizations will be taken over by the ego and made into an ego agenda. Spiritual community can also support individuals through times of difficulty, confusion, or loss of resolve. Although expressed with different language across spiritual traditions, these three themes of the possibility of enlightenment, harmonious living revealed through contemplation in community, and contemplative spiritual community as material aid and as protection against contamination by self-centered motives, are present in most widespread religious traditions that have stood the test of time.

LIFE STAGES AND SPIRITUAL DEVELOPMENT

Although some early theories linked spiritual development to the demands of sociocultural life stages, life stages evolve, and the number of life stages, especially in later life, has increased in recent years. In the 1950s, when Erikson was developing his theory, the dominant view was that after age 65 people experienced just one life stage—old age. In the late 1960s, Bernice Neugarten began to write about the young-old (65–74) and the old-old (75 and older). By the early 1970s, gerontologists were talking about the young-old (65–74), middle-old (75–84), and old-old (85 and older). In 2004, I was writing about the nearly-old (55–64), young-old (65–74), middle-old (75–84), older-old (85–94), and oldest-old (95 and older). By 2015, I suspect that I will be splitting those 95 and older into the oldest-old (95–104) and the hyper-old (105 and older). The point here is that the population of interest in research on aging contains a span of more than fifty years in terms of chronological age. Breaking this population into ten-year categories gives us the ability to compare people approaching or at the beginning of later life with people who are farther along in the age range.

Richard Settersten (2003) drew attention to a growing gap between the concept of a culturally given set of life stages and the concept of the human life course as an individual life path conditioned by decisions and circumstances in response not only to life stage but also to current events, personal preferences, subcultural worldviews, and a host of other factors. Indeed, there is a great deal of support for the existence of abstract notions of life stages, such as middle age and old age (Atchley and Barusch 2004), but when researchers tried to ascertain details of these conceptions, such as when life stage transitions begin or end, or how social expectations change from one life stage to another, or even how many life stages there are, they came away confused (Settersten 1999). This suggests that, like spirituality, life stage is a sensitizing concept that takes you only to a general area of interest, one with only general dimensions. The particulars have to be investigated for each emerging life stage.

For our present purposes, is there spiritual development unique to those who live to advanced old age, say those over 100? I would expect so, but so far there has been little study of this aspect of centenarians. If we think about these admittedly arbitrary lifestage divisions of the age range in later life, do people in these various life stages expect different things of themselves in terms of spirituality? Does the community expect different things from them in terms of qualities such as spiritual wisdom? How might these differing expectations influence the experience of spiritual development? These are just a few of the possible research questions as we chart the new territory of having large numbers of people survive to very advanced old age. The difficulty of addressing these questions is compounded by our cultural inability to agree about labels and definitions of the life stages past age 80.

CONCLUSION

This chapter begins with a history of the study of spiritual development since the 1950s and presents several different approaches to understanding how spiritual capacity in an individual evolves over time, what stimulates spiritual development, and how spiritual development interacts with other aspects of adult development.

Erikson's theory presumes that spiritual development is built on a resolution of the successive developmental challenges associated with each stage of life before middle age. For Erikson, spiritual development begins in middle age with a development of generativity—a concern for the well-being of younger generations—and in later adulthood grows to include wisdom and gerotranscendence. To Erikson, changes in social expectations associated with later life stages couple nicely with inner predispositions toward a spiritual rather than a personal "I" and a metaperspective called gerotranscendence. For Tornstam, gerotranscendence is an intrinsic process that social circumstances can only hinder. Tornstam sees gerotranscendence as being present to some extent in all aging people and as having cosmic, self-transcendent, and social selectivity elements.

Moody and Carroll present a linear theory of spiritual development as a progression through five stages: call, search, struggle, breakthrough, and return. Moody and Carroll use these stages mainly to describe large changes in engagement with one's spirituality over an extended period of time. I use a similar series of phases to describe smaller, short-term *cycles* of spiritual development: awakening interest, inquiry, endeavor, integration, and intention.

Wilber developed what is probably the most ambitious and complex theory of spiritual development to date. He sees spiritual development evolving along multiple lines and through several levels of consciousness. Unfortunately, his theory has not been applied to the issues of adult development and aging.

Ray and McFadden see spiritual development as involving a necessary element of human relationship. Their concept of development is not so much a linear or even cyclic process. They prefer the web and the quilt as metaphors for the mysterious interactive processes by which disparate spiritual experiences result in a meaningful spiritual whole.

These examples of conceptualizing and theorizing about spiritual development by no means exhaust the possibilities, but they amply illustrate that each perspective contains valuable insights. There is no need to pick one as "truth" and junk the rest. Rather, it is possible to integrate all these perspectives into a more complete understanding of spiritual development as an important possibility in later adulthood.

Now, let us turn to the relation among spirituality, spiritual development, and identity and the self.

CHAPTER THREE

Spirituality, Spiritual Self, and Spiritual Identity

What is my spiritual nature? How do I develop spiritually? These were the basic questions addressed in the two previous chapters. The basic question for this chapter is, How does spirituality influence identity and self, and vice versa? How do I experience myself, conceive of myself, and aspire for myself, and how does spiritual experience interact with these elements? Where does spirituality reside in my holistic conception of self?

To deal with these issues, we must first have a good sense of what we mean by the terms *identity* and *self*. Then we can look at how these concepts relate to spiritual experience and ideas. We also look at continuity theory as a framework for understanding how spiritual identity and self are developed and adapted to a constantly changing personal and social environment.

CONCEPTS ABOUT THE SELF AND IDENTITY

The self has two different aspects. The first is *self as experiencer*, which consists of awareness of being and witness of self as actor—self as the doer, the feeler of emotions, and the feeler of motivation. Both awareness of being and perception of acting can happen without reflective thought and without words. But as soon as we begin to think about the content of various dimensions of self—to conceptualize, categorize, and interpret them—a second aspect of self arises—the *reflective self*. The noted sociologist G. H. Mead referred to the first self as the "I" and the second as the "Me." The I consists of bare experience of being: "I am," which we earlier equated with basic spirituality, and experience of self as the center of action: "I do," "I feel," "I want." The Me is a much more complicated system of thoughts about oneself, which come both from the person's own perceptions of self (what C. H. Cooley called the "looking-glass self") and from messages about the self that come from others, called "reflected appraisals" based on how we perceive others' reactions to us and our behavior.[1]

Thoughts about the self can be divided into *self-concept* (what I think I am actually like), *ideal self* (what I think I should be like), *feared self* (the self I am afraid I might become), *self-evaluation* (my assessment of the fit between actual and ideal self), and *self-esteem* (how much I like or dislike myself, often based on my self-evaluation). Self-concept can be further differentiated into more detailed concepts, such as *self-confidence*, or willingness to act, which incorporates an element of agency into the self. Another term for *agency* is *self-efficacy*, an expectation that my efforts will be successful. *Self-acceptance* is a process that can involve increasing acceptance of the actual self by letting go of a perfectionistic ideal self in favor or a more realistic ideal, thereby increasing self-esteem. In all this, the I as actor takes an active part in constructing and maintaining the self system, even when the result is a confused self-concept, unclear ideal self, negative self-evaluation, and poor self-esteem.

The *self system* is a dynamic collection of self-referential ideas and a process for creating and maintaining the system through feedback from life experience. By observing the self in action, people develop *self-schemas* such as "I am a spiritual person," "I am an honest person," "I am a loner," "I am a good guitar player," "I am a frail old man," "I have a mean streak," or "I work well with people." "The domains of individuals' self-schemas reflect what they think about, what they care about, and what they spend their time and energy on" (Markus and Herzog 1991, 113). Self-schemas serve as benchmarks for evaluating and refining the self in the context of current life experience. In addition, people have scenarios about "possible selves" they could become. In actively constructing an ideal self of the future, people use their ideas about hoped-for or feared possible selves (Markus and Nurius 1986).

In psychoanalytic terms, the psyche includes a self that has both conscious and unconscious or nonconscious elements. Carl Jung's analytical psychology emphasizes, among many other things, the importance of bringing aspects of the self that exist in the unconscious into consciousness.[2] This cannot be done directly, says Jung, but it can be done through the use of metaphors and myths, through interpretation of dreams, and through art (Jung and Jaffe 1962). The art people make is an important research tool in accessing their understandings about the self that reside outside their verbal, conceptual mind.

Moody (unpublished) recounts the following dream:

I dreamed that I was in a subway station, on the platform. Built into the wall were bookcases filled with books, very impressive looking (gilded, antique, heavily bound). But when I examined some of the books, perhaps to buy them, I discovered that the pages were empty, that the books were high-class trash, [empty pages] dressed up to look good. Then I was sitting in a row of spiritual seekers on one side of the platform. I recognized two friends among them. Across the tracks, alone on the other side, sitting on a kind of throne was a great spiritual master. He answered a question from one of my friends, and his answer made it clear that the Way did not mean getting rid of anything with intellectual value; that is, we should not be anti-intellectual. I felt this was somehow a message for me.

Moody goes on to interpret this dream.

The "subway station" here is a place below ground, a path for traveling into the Underworld, or the depths of the self. The opening imagery of the dream is of bookcases filled with marvelous books. As an academic, I would naturally be attracted by such beautiful books displayed down in this lower world. But in this dream I discover that the books are all empty, suggesting that purely intellectual knowledge has nothing [to offer the spiritual struggle]. As a wise man once remarked to me while I sat carefully reading the menu at a restaurant, "You could read this menu all night and you would still be hungry." Yet the message of this dream is not entirely a repudiation of the intellect, as if intelligence were an evil to be overcome, as certain religious traditions suggest; for example, when faith is opposed to reason. Instead, the dreamer hears a message from a spiritual master who helps him overcome any dualism.

Moody's dream exposed the dilemma of his shadow anti-intellectual self and his academic self and showed a way to integrate them.

To Jung, the "shadow self" is an unconscious aspect of self comprising suppressed aspects of self. The shadow self can be destructive or constructive. The destructive shadow is made up of negative self-referential observations that the individual actively disowns or does not want to acknowledge. None of us likes to admit negative qualities such as unkindness, dishonesty, cruelty, and the like. On the other hand, the constructive shadow is made up of potentially positive attributes of self that go unacknowledged for a variety of

SPIRITUALITY, SPIRITUAL SELF, AND SPIRITUAL IDENTITY   49

reasons. For instance, many people have spiritual experiences but deny them because of their *belief* that spirituality does not exist.

Both Erikson and Jung agree that healthy development requires that we face our "negative" or disvalued qualities and learn to accept them. Erikson called this kind of self-acceptance *integrity* and saw it as a central developmental task of old age. Likewise, if spiritual growth is to be a possibility, the individual must be open to that aspect of self.

It is often said that the complexity of language about a subject is a clue to its importance. *Webster's Dictionary* (Agnes 2002) listed more than a hundred words describing different aspects of the personal self. The scores of terms and concepts for various aspects of self show that the self is of great interest to most people, and most of us spend a lot of time thinking and talking about ourselves.

Because the self-system in most people is open to change stimulated by life experience, spiritual experiences—especially if they are cumulative—can have profound effects on all the elements of self described thus far. Spiritual experiences and development can be a major force in the shift from a concrete, mechanistic view of self to a more dynamic, open approach. In *The Presentation of Self in Everyday Life*, Erving Goffman (1959) popularized the notion that, because reflected appraisals from others are so important, we spend a great deal of energy trying to manipulate others' appraisals of us by tweaking our presentation of self. Like stage actors, we take on costumes and personas to created illusions that we think will be attractive to others. This perspective may well be important for explaining motives and behavior of adolescents and young adults, but by middle age, most people's life experience has suggested that such manipulation is not an effective route to acceptance by others of the actual self and that presenting an inauthentic self is a trap that one can become caught in. Likewise, many changes associated with aging require some modification if the self is to remain relevant and adaptive to current life circumstances. For example, taking advantage of the opportunity for a more humane pace of life in retirement often requires letting go of the "productive" ideal self, with its perfectionism and potential inappropriateness to the spiritual goals of later adulthood.

CONTINUITY THEORY AND THE SELF

Continuity theory (Atchley 1999) is a useful framework for exploring the interchange between spirituality and self and identity over the life course.

Continuity theory was created to explain evolutionary human development. It is an open-feedback-systems theory, which means that it starts from the assumption that systems are created to meet needs and are modified to take into account feedback from the results of using the systems. In this chapter, the self system is the system of primary interest.[3]Why do we need a self system? If we look at life as improvisational theater, then the satisfaction we can get from our social performance may depend on knowing what character we are playing. How do we know our character?

Identity is the unique set of characteristics and qualities considered collectively and regarded as essential to a person's self-awareness. In other words, identity is a holistic self-concept, a sort of metaconception of self created by synthesizing multitudes of specific attributes, capabilities, life experiences, motives, habits, and preferences. James Hillman (1999) uses the word *character* to refer to an individual's creative description of self. To Hillman, character stresses the uniqueness and singularity of each person. A dramaturgical metaphor is again helpful: much can happen to a character in a play, but throughout the play that character is still identifiably different from other characters. This illustrates the holistic quality of character and identity and the importance of continuity for a subjective sense of being "in character."

According to Hillman, character is a celebration of the unique psychosomatic being we call a person. Character is descriptive detail. Character is not unified into a closely integrated whole but instead looks like a loosely wound core with lots of loose ends. Character reveals itself not in the morality of behavior but in its style. Character is an imaginative description, and the self perceives its character in a context involving other characters in a setting. Character gives sense and purpose to the changes of aging, according to Hillman.

A major question for us is how spirituality manifests itself in character. Character development involves making decisions that stress certain attributes and capacities and downplay or ignore other attributes or capacities. So where does spirituality fit into character in young adulthood compared with middle age and later adulthood? What aspirations or fears lead to deepening the spiritual aspects of character or to suppressing them?

Abraham Maslow (1968) considered *self-actualization* to be the highest human need. Once basic physiological, safety, belonging, and esteem needs have been met, an individual can be motivated toward "growth" needs such as spirituality, creativity, and transcendence. Malsow's theory of human self-motivation, with its assumption that, once free of the grind of basic needs, people strive to make the most of their capacities and be the best they can be, was a lynchpin of the human potential movement. Maslow's theory presumes that character is already there in the bud, just waiting to bloom. Hillman says that the freedom from social constraints that often comes with aging creates conditions for increasingly becoming who you already are. Implicit in Hillman's conception of self-actualization is increasing self-acceptance—a willingness to make friends with one's disvalued as well as valued character, one's feared as well as hoped-for character. For many people, spirituality is an increasingly important aspect of character that is both realized and hoped for.

Development of the self is continuous, and evolution of the self occurs mainly through small, incremental changes rather than through cataclysmic crises. By the time most people are in their 40s, they have a well-developed and highly refined self system that has been tested thousands of times. A large majority of middle-aged and older people have a self system that provides positive life satisfaction and self-esteem, but those who have created, or had imposed on them, a system that provides poor life satisfaction and low self-esteem have a heavy weight to lift if they wish to change. One way to lift such a burden is through religious conversion, which, if genuine, suddenly makes major changes in all of the elements of the self—self-concept, ideal self, self-evaluation, and self-esteem.

CONTINUITY OF ONE'S SELF SYSTEM

Consider the following story.

> At age 6, Jenny enjoys the experience of singing—she loves the sound she makes and the feeling of vibration in her chest when she sings. She is told by many people that she has a nice voice. She chooses singing every chance she gets. In middle school, she sings in the school choir and in the youth choir at her church. She takes voice lessons an hour each week. When Jenny sings, especially in the church choir, she often has an experience of being in an altered, expanded state. She "loses herself" in the music.
>
> By high school, Jenny has a solid and well-confirmed concept of herself as a good singer. She not only sings in various choirs and in amateur stage productions, she has learned to play the guitar and is learning to write her own songs, mostly about everyday experiences. In college, she no longer has the time to sing in multiple choirs and does not attend

church anymore, but she continues to perform her songs in coffee houses and local bars, partly for the joy of performing, partly for the money, and partly for the applause and recognition. She records an album of her songs that enjoys good sales locally. Jenny dreams of being a famous singer. After college, she tries to make a career of singing and songwriting, but it is a difficult life with lots of rejections and financial difficulty. She goes back to school to get a master's degree in social work. She works with girls who are first-time offenders in the juvenile justice system. She continues to sing in various local venues, usually once a week.

At 28, Jenny marries and continues to work. She cuts her performing back to once a month. By 34, she has two children, and soon she is teaching her two girls to make up songs with titles like "Sharon wears purple shoes." When she performs now, her husband and kids are usually in the audience, which means she only does coffee houses that have an early show and sings more songs that kids might enjoy. Turns out most adults enjoy those songs too. Jenny records an album of her own songs for children.

When Jenny is 45, the kids are "doing their own thing" and Jenny has been promoted to director of her program. Her husband travels a lot in his work, but they enjoy long family vacations about three times a year. She always takes her guitar on their vacations and there is much group singing. She also sings a lot as she drives alone from this to that. She still performs occasionally but not often enough to maintain a local following.

At 57, Jenny has kids in college. Her agency "reorganizes" to eliminate the program she directs and she faces a reassignment that essentially means starting over. She is eligible to retire, so she does. Almost immediately, Jenny begins writing songs again and performing more often. Within a year she begins volunteering twice a week teaching music in an after-school program for middle school students. She joins a local choir that sings mostly classical religious music and she rediscovers the classical voice she worked so hard to create in high school. She also rediscovers the feeling of transcendence that can come to her while singing. Jenny also joins a group of mostly older folk singers who get together for a once-a-month sing-along.

Jenny says that she only recently consciously realized that music is her spiritual path. She does not consider herself religious but considers herself a spiritual person.

Jenny's story is an abbreviated version of one thread in her rich life, the interplay between her experience of music—the satisfaction, spiritual experience, and social recognition music brings, and how this aspect of her self has been involved in her decision making thus far in her life. Would we expect music to play a role in Jenny's life when she's in her 70s? Yes. Why? Continuity theory.

Continuity theory holds that people develop mental frameworks based on life experience (Jenny's early perceptions that music brought her many satisfactions), make decisions based on them (Jenny's continuing to choose music over other possible activities), observe the results and modify the frameworks to improve them (Jenny's dropping the idea of music as a way of earning a living), and continue to make decisions and adapt their frameworks (Jenny's adapting her music to fit the circumstances of her life at each stage). Creating a self system constitutes a substantial investment of time and energy that people become increasingly reluctant to abandon as they age. This reluctance is usually not based in fear but in the potential for joy and satisfaction that continuity represents to the person. Continuity theory offers clues about why people take specific directions and how they adapt to life events. It is also a model of how people learn from their life experience.

How people process feedback is at the heart of continuity theory. Psychologist George Kelly (1955) created *personal construct psychology* based on his observation that people do not share exactly the same meanings for the language they use in thinking. Each word we use has our own unique set of images, feelings, and life experiences attached to it. This is especially true of the abstract language we use in analytical thought. This means that each person has a unique, personal language he or she uses to organize, categorize, analyze, and summarize perceptions, including perceptions of spirituality, identity, and self.

Other important elements of processing feedback include attentional and observational skills. By paying attention and observing skillfully, we obtain better information to feed back into the personal construct system we have created concerning the self. Each choice we make has results that, if we are paying attention and carefully observing, we can use to refine our ideas about the self to make them more useful and, with age, usually more realistic.

Continuity theory has two important implications for research. First, there is no standard "template" for the self systems people create; each system is based on the individual's life experiences, awareness skills, and personal constructs. Research must therefore begin by investigating the individual's vocabulary about the self. Second, to understand the evolution of identity and self requires longitudinal information. To understand how a person's self system evolves, we must observe it at different points in time, because retrospective reports are notoriously revisionist (Greenwald 1980). What people revise is important information about the self they want to construct. In a research world heavily committed to standardized survey language, continuity theory requires that researchers acknowledge and accommodate individual language and life experience, which increases the complexity and expense of research.

Now let us consider how spiritual experience, including thoughts about spiritual aspects of life, influences various aspects of self and identity, and vice versa. Given what I discussed about spiritual development in the previous chapter, it is important to consider spirituality as a possible influence in development from early in life.

SPIRITUAL SELF-SCHEMAS AND SPIRITUAL IDENTITY

Observing how individuals respond to the following self-referential statements is an effective way to ascertain an individual's spiritual self-schemas and identity. Each statement asserts a relation between spirituality and self or identity.

I am a person who has spiritual experiences.

Individuals who agree with this statement are acknowledging that spiritual experiences are possible and that they have spiritual experiences. This is the most basic form of incorporating spirituality into the self concept. Spiritual experiences can be at the being level and at the perceiving level. For example, "I was aware of enormous space within me" or "I looked into his eyes and saw a being just like me."

Personal constructs are used to define experiences as spiritual. Say I have an experience of being pleasantly detached from my physical body. How do I interpret this experience? Is it evidence of mental illness? Is it a reflection of the existence of a spiritual level of consciousness beyond what I am normally aware of? Is it just a temporary aberration with no meaning? What I am predisposed to think about such experiences profoundly influences how I interpret them. What I am predisposed to think about spiritual experiences is deeply conditioned by the concepts, language, and customs I learned through socialization to a specific ethnic and social class culture, which also includes several specific religious cultures. But the influence of culture is also mediated by my personal worldview, my central personal constructs.

When spiritual experiences are converted into thoughts about the Me, they become part of the objectified self. For most people, it is difficult to have an experience without thinking at some level "This is happening to *me*." As we saw earlier, many different types of experience can be classified as spiritual, and by the time people reach adulthood most have a substantial number of spiritual experiences tucked away in memory.

Spiritual teachings and teachers point the way and also provide mental, linguistic frameworks for organizing our spiritual experiences. Rick Moody relates the story of his interview with Jeffrey:

> One day Jeffrey met a Sufi teacher at a friend's apartment. At the time, he explained, Islam conjured up the usual stereotypes of sword-wielding Arabs and terrorists at the airport. Meeting this elderly Sufi changed all that.
>
> "I sort of had . . . well, when I first met him my heart exploded in me. I felt like I'd always known this man; always wanted to be with him. Something like that—it's hard to describe these things."
>
> At the request of his teacher, Jeffrey converted to Islam. "I didn't know anything about Islam, but one passage of the Koran got me: "Wheresoever you look, there is the face of God."
>
> Moody pressed Jeffrey for guidance that might lead Moody to have a similar experience.
>
> "You know, seeing God isn't for everyone," Jeffrey said. "In Sufism we talk about a person's heart being open. People assume that this is the goal, that all of us have to get to this place. But it isn't true.
>
> "The reason for being on a path is not always to have 'experiences.' You struggle spiritually because that's what you're put on earth to do. It's your job as a human being. Whether or not you get to the light is not what matters. If you do, great. If you don't, great. We can't really understand how it works. It just happens to some people and not to others. That's another reason why it's better not to talk about it—it makes people feel badly that they haven't experienced what you've experienced. Better to just keep it to yourself."
>
> Jeffrey's statement reminded [Moody] of a Sufi saying: "The more one talks about their vision of God, the faster you should run away."
>
> Jeffrey went on, "If your heart opens and you see light or angels, or whatever, afterward when it's over you feel small and invisible. You realize you didn't do anything; you didn't really make the thing happen. It was given to you, and that's all you can say about it."
>
> When asked "What should one do, then?" Jeffrey said, "Small things. Start with small things. Efforts that are within your power. Everyday efforts

to be nice to somebody, to be patient. Try to see the matter from the other guy's point of view. Try to understand that maybe this person is having a bad day. Be generous. Give away something you like to someone who needs it. Be cheerful when you're not feeling so good. . . . Try not to make things into tragedies if you can help it. Little things.

"Let me say something else. Most of us are easily distracted. We're pulled along by the current of things. But, you know, if you want to become an accountant you don't study law one year, art the next, medicine the next. You'd never make it that way. You have to make a commitment. Choose something and stay with it. It's the same with spiritual things. . . . A person has to go at this with deep sincerity. . . . The commitment is what's important. Let the rest take care of itself." (Adapted from Moody and Carroll, 1997: 304–8)

Moody's experience of Jeffrey reveals important elements about spiritual teachers. First, Jeffrey provided a conceptual overview of the nature of the spiritual journey and language that Moody could use to interpret his own spiritual experiences. Second, there was something about Jeffrey that led Moody to perceive what Jeffrey was saying as authentic. Jeffrey himself embodied for Moody what Jeffrey was teaching.

I feel separated or alienated from my spiritual self.

In his book, *A Hidden Wholeness*, Parker Palmer (2004) describes a self divided from soul: "We lose touch with our souls—the core of pure being that children are so intimate with—and disappear into our roles" (15). The result is a compartmentalized life in which the core self is somewhat alienated from each of the compartmentalized selves because each compartment requires that we deny other parts of the self. Palmer feels that "a divided life may be endemic, but wholeness is always a choice" (17).

Palmer believes that the "true self" is powerful, real, and spiritual, but shy.

Just like a wild animal . . . [the true self] seeks safety in the dense under-brush, especially when other people are around. If we want to see a wild animal, we know that the last thing we should do is go crashing through the woods yelling for it to come out. But if we will walk quietly into the woods, sit patiently at the base of a tree, breathe with the earth, and fade into our surroundings, the wild creature we seek might put in an appearance. We may see it only briefly and only out of the corner of an eye—but the sight is a gift we will always treasure as an end in itself. (58–59)

For Palmer, the spiritual journey is a journey of reuniting soul and role.

In Zen Buddhism, the spiritual quest is sometimes depicted as "the search for an elusive Ox that roams wild in the rain forest. The Ox symbolizes the intrinsic nature of consciousness, the mystery of what we are" (Hixon 1978, 77). Having turned his back on his true nature, the man cannot see the Ox. He has lost sight of it but still he feels a need to search. The progression of the spiritual journey is shown in a series of ten "Zen Ox-herding pictures": seeking the Ox, finding the tracks, first glimpse of the Ox, catching the Ox, taming the Ox, riding the Ox home, Ox forgotten-self alone, both Ox and self forgotten, return to the source, and entering the marketplace with helping hands (figures 1–10). Note that once more metaphor points the way to realities that are difficult to express in discursive language.

Rick Moody tells the following story about himself.

> I am not one person inside, but two. The first is a highly social being who sits in an office in Manhattan all day, talks on the phone to colleagues around the country, writes scholarly papers, delivers lectures, directs workshops, jokes, argues, gives orders and advice, and at home kicks the soccer ball around with his son. A pillar of the community. That's the visible [Rick] Moody in the external world.
>
> Beneath this outer mask, however, lives an entirely different being with roots deeply sunk into the invisible. This second being is a rather gentle, passive soul, a good deal quieter than the erudite professor who goes to the office every day, and a good deal closer to the center of reality. I have caught phantom glimpses of him through the years, sometimes in the midst of ordinary activities, most often during meditation. . . . This self remains so remote and silent that at times I wonder why it's there at all. If the soul doesn't play a part in everyday life, what part does it play? Surely this soul has important lessons to contribute. . . . Why then does it sit so passively in the shadows of our consciousness, often unheard and unacknowledged throughout out lives?
>
> The answer is that it is not sitting there passively. It is actually calling to us all the time, sending us message after message. . . . But it is doing so in its own secret language, the language of spiritual communication—symbol, contemplation, art, ceremony, and especially our dreams. (adapted from Moody and Carroll 1997, 51–52)

This applies mainly to self as experiencer, the "I am." Moody is in direct contact with his spiritual self and has integrated that self with his conventional social self.

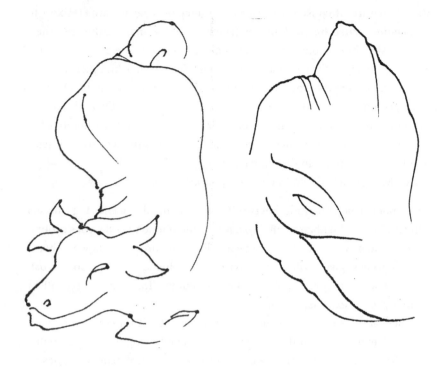

Figure 1. Seeking the ox. "The Ox has really never gone astray. Our True Nature is never lost and therefore can never be found" (Hixon 1978, 88).

Figure 2. Finding the tracks. "These tracks are the wisdom teaching that all phenomena are the light of Original Mind. Even the deepest gorges or the topmost mountains cannot hide this Ox's nose, which reaches right to Heaven" (Hixon 1978, 89).

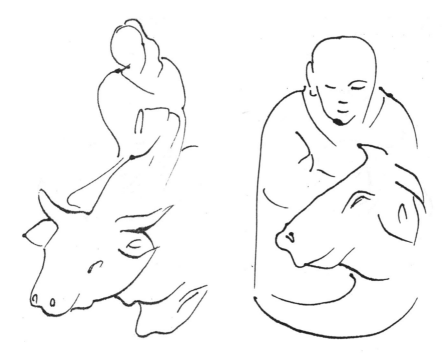

Figure 3. First glimpse of the ox. "This encounter with the Ox does not come through hearing esoteric teaching but through direct experience" (Hixon 1978, 90).

Figure 4. Catching the ox. "We must now hold and embrace the Ox, sustain our perception of True Nature with such disciplines as total compassion, perfect nonviolence, unwavering truthfulness" (Hixon 1978, 91).

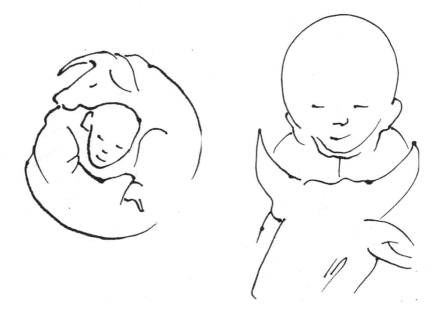

Figure 5. Taming the ox. "An effortless intimacy or friendship with the Ox is being established. The Ox becomes a free companion, not a tool for plowing the field of Enlightenment" (Hixon 1978, 92).

Figure 6. Riding the ox home. "The advanced practitioner now becomes the illumined sage. The struggle is over. The sage begins spontaneously to radiate enlightenment" (Hixon 1978, 93).

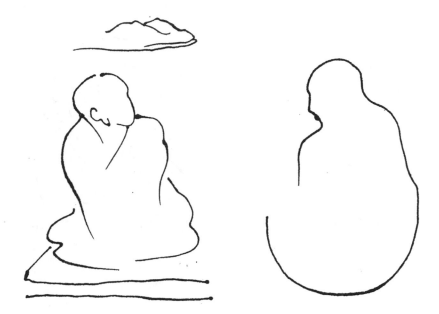

Figure 7. Ox forgotten, self alone. "The sage finally regards [him/her] self as the full expression of True Nature. All spiritual practices and concepts are idle. The contemplative way has become indistinguishable from daily life" (Hixon 1978, 94).

Figure 8. Both ox and self forgotten. "There is only awakened Enlightenment: no contemplator and no contemplation, no serenity and no disturbance. There is no one, not even the sage" (Hixon 1978, 95).

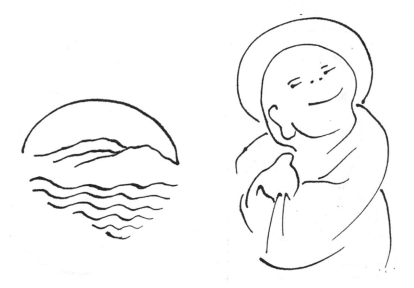

Figure 9. Return to the source. "Formless awareness is growing back into form again without losing its formless, or perfectly unitary, nature. Enlightenment simply *is* the blue lake and the green mountain" (Hixon 1978, 96).

Figure 10. Entering the marketplace with helping hands. "The cheerful one who fully manifests Enlightenment follows no path" (Hixon 1978, 97). He or she sees the world as it is and understands what compassionate action or inaction is appropriate to each moment.

William James wrote,

> One may say truly, I think, that personal religious experience has its roots and center in mystical states of consciousness. . . . Our normal waking consciousness, rational consciousness we call it, is but one special type of consciousness, while all about it, parted from it by the filmiest of screens, there lie potential forms of consciousness entirely different. We may go through life without suspecting their existence; but apply the requisite stimulus, and at a touch they are there in all their completeness . . . No account of the universe in its totality can be final which leaves these other forms of consciousness quite disregarded. How to regard them is the question. (James [1905] 2005, 313)

The literature on spirituality contains many and varied accounts of a true or core spiritual self from which humans tend to become separated. The accounts above give some sense of the range of language, concepts, and images that have been used to address this issue.

I am a spiritual person.

Spirituality shifts from being a category of ordinary experiences to being a self-defining category, part of identity. In my longitudinal study of people who were age 70 or older in 1996 (Atchley 1999) only about 30 percent saw themselves as spiritual persons. In Wade Roof's (1999) study of individuals who were in their 40s in 1988, a large majority saw themselves as spiritual, and this proportion increased over time, to 73 percent in 1998. Zinnbauer et al. (1997) reported that 93 percent of their respondents rated themselves as spiritual persons. George Gallup (2003) reported that in 2002, 47 percent of a national sample "strongly agreed" with the statement "I am a person who is spiritually committed," and the proportion with spiritual commitment increased with age. These findings suggest that the growing use of the term *spiritual* to describe inner experiences of being and transcendence took hold more for those who had come of age in the 1950s and that for many there was also a developmental shift toward seeing oneself as a spiritual person as one aged.

What are the implications of spirituality becoming part of identity? It seems reasonable to suspect that it becomes harder to relegate spirituality to one or two compartments of lifestyle and that spirituality identity might be expected to influence how a person approaches life in many more contexts.

I feel attracted, drawn, or called to a spiritual journey.

Something happens to create an opening, an invitation that may come in many forms: an experience that suggests we are not who we thought we were, feeling homesick for a place we don't recall being before, or an experience of an alternative universe in our consciousness. Ron's story illustrates how our perspective can suddenly be shifted by a single life experience.

Ron attended a leadership training workshop for student affairs workers from many colleges. He knew only a couple of the 150 people there, and none of them was in his small group. On the beginning evening of the workshop, each small group of 10 people was given the task of doing a group painting. It was a pleasant enough task, but Ron felt that he didn't know much more about the people in his group when the task was completed than he had before, which was nothing.

The next morning, the small groups were asked to fill out a form for each person in their small group, rating them on a series of personal qualities, both positive and negative. Then the group was to pick a person to start with, discuss that person's qualities and come to consensus about them, and then move on to the next person until everyone had been discussed. The person being discussed was to remain in the room but could not speak while he or she was being discussed.

The group selected Ron as the first focus person, and for the entire three hours allotted to this task, Ron listened in growing amazement as this group of people with little experience of Ron argued about what Ron was like. At first, Ron was disturbed by the vehemence of the negative comments, but the longer the polarized discussion went on, the more detached he felt. At some point he had a deep realization: "What these strangers see when they look at me has little to do with me, what I think or do, my personal qualities, nothing. I am like an empty screen and they are quite willing to project their own preconceptions onto it." Ron felt liberated by this discussion, liberated from what he had seen as a need to conform to his "role." He began to look into himself to see what he was really like, to reconcile the inner man with the outer, to be more authentic in an existential, real sense. Ron sees this experience as the beginning of his spiritual journey.

Until this point, Ron had focused his self system on the feedback he received from others and had paid less attention to his own inner voice. After this experience, he saw firsthand the limitations and unreliability of others' appraisals as a guide for his development and for his own clarity of self-awareness. He became motivated to more consciously examine his inner self, the "I am."

One of the great mysteries is why some people see such experiences as an invitation to a spiritual journey and others do not. My impression is that this probably relates to what the person is paying attention to and how open he or she is to the possibility of a spiritual journey.

I am a person on a spiritual journey. I am a spiritual seeker.

A spiritual journey is an exploration—"evolving, open-ended, and revisable" (Roof 1999, 78). Wade Roof followed a panel of several hundred respondents through the early part of middle age and found that "there was a remarkable degree of clarity about themselves as [being] engaged in a process-oriented spirituality and what that engagement may involve for them. Reflexive spirituality is not haphazard or left to chance; it seeks self-understanding and self-management" (102). Saying that one is on a spiritual journey is a statement of commitment. As mentioned earlier, Gallup (2003) found that 47 percent of a national sample of adults saw themselves as "spiritually committed." Roof's respondents who were on a spiritual journey were likely to stick with it. The journey usually starts with mysterious inner forces, but *the individual* makes the decisions about which forks in the road to take and how to monitor results, although others may attempt to influence these decisions. Along the way, most people make choices that balance the need for openness and the need for group support and security. Most people on a spiritual journey create a narrative about it. "This story provides a way for them to understand their origins, how they have changed, and the role that crisis events or significant others have played in their lives, and where they think they are headed" (Wuthnow 1998, 186). Robert Wuthnow adds that the self-directed spiritual journey is both liberating and scary because it requires "people to do more of the work needed to understand spirituality and to put it into practice" (13–14). Roof (1999) reported that the 60 percent of his respondents who saw themselves as being on a spiritual journey came from every sort of religious background, including evangelical and conservative Christian.

There are three major patterns of spiritual journey (Roof 1999). The first pattern involves assimilating and conforming to a religious culture and gradually integrating this culture into one's own personal constructs. Individuals who choose this pattern enjoy the security of knowing what to expect and tolerate well the constraints their religion requires. Even in this pattern, however, individuals usually see themselves as responsible for the specific elements of the journey. The second pattern is an individualized journey within a religious context. It often involves clergy as personal counselors who help the individual integrate religious beliefs and practices with personal constructs of meaning and purpose. The third pattern is the self-directed spiritual journey. Individuals following this pattern may use free-lance "spiritual directors" to help them gain the self-awareness and make the decisions needed to fashion, maintain, and revise their spiritual journey. Others are comfortable being on their own in searching, selecting, and processing feedback from experience on the spiritual journey.

Seeing oneself as a *seeker*, a person who is actively pursuing and cultivating spiritual experience and integrating those experiences into her or his life, is not a concept that all people on a spiritual journey would apply to themselves. Seekers are more actively searching and choosing and learning and applying. In Moody and Carroll's (1996) terms, we would expect seeking to be an early phase of spiritual development, followed by settling into a meaningful spiritual routine.

I am a person on a particular spiritual path.

In Hinduism, people speak of many yogas, or ways, of spiritual knowing: understanding, good works, devotion, body movement, and breathing. Study, contemplation, devotional practice, and service to others are main ways the self can manifest spirituality in the world in most major spiritual traditions. But in our postmodern world, the multiplicity of pathways can be daunting. Within each spiritual tradition, there are numerous combinations of injunction and technique, and individuals can get stuck at the point of making a commitment about which paths to try. A person who needs to look at all the shoes in the store before trying on a pair may never get to the point of trying on any. Roof (1999) found that most respondents who were on a spiritual journey had settled into a routine practice by the ten-year follow-up. I have found that descriptions of the spiritual path are highly individualistic, tailored to fit the personal constructs, life opportunities, and background of the person. The highly individualized nature of spiritual paths is also evident in the many case studies reported by Moody and Carroll (1996), Wuthnow (1998), and Roof (1999).

I have had an experience of spiritual transformation.

People who agree with this statement have personal experiences of being transformed spiritually from one state or level to another. A 2002 Gallup Poll found that 41 percent of adults said the statement "I have had a profound awakening that changed the direction of my life" applied to them completely (Gallup 2003).

To Ken Wilber (2006), transformation occurs when we leave behind an old structure and embrace a new one. So when we leave behind an old spiritual worldview and adopt a new one, we have been transformed. Spiritual transformations sometimes occur in response to a dramatic experience: a near-death experience, the collapse of the previous worldview in the face of feedback, a response to the charisma of a teacher or teaching, a sudden religious conversion. Transformation is not just an incremental improvement or rearrangement of ideas but a fundamental restructuring of the way we see things. Wilber says that transformation involves transcending a previous structure, but including it. The previous self does not disappear; it is included as a set of resources the new self has available. So when we are transformed, we do not forget how to love our children, drive a car, or do our income taxes. We may leave behind old habits, but we still know we had them in the past. We simply see all that has gone before in an entirely different context. The "include" part of Wilber's "transcend and include" framework is important because if we deny or repress our past, it remains as a shadow self, not open to reflection. Including all of one's previous stages in one's self system is essential to what Wilber calls "integral spirituality."

Moody and Carroll (1997, 272–73) list several attributes of transformational experiences, which they call "breakthroughs": a perception of timelessness and "placelessness"—a person feels as if the ordinary world with its boundaries and limitations is dissolved or at least deeply altered; a conviction that the breakthrough experience reveals a world much closer to "reality" than was possible in one's previous state of consciousness; a new sense of liberation, freedom, and lightness—the weight of the world becomes easier to bear; perceptions of light, serenity, and universal love; loss of fears about death; feelings of renewal and new beginnings—some speak of "rebirth"; and a clear perception that this transformation experience cannot be "adequately expressed in ordinary language." Many people use the expression "coming home" to describe their spiritual transformation. Many people I've interviewed report that after experiencing a spiritual transformation, events and lessons that in the past seemed confusing or unclear become clear. Many people react with amusement at their previous "denseness." Moody and Carroll (1997, 273) write, "Breakthroughs may seem to occur suddenly and seemingly out of the blue. In reality, these moments usually come after many years of daily struggle and time spent in care of the soul."

Many people feel that because they have been transformed, their troubles ought to be over. A transformed perspective can certainly provide greater detachment from the personality and its foibles, but the personality does not disappear. Thus, spiritual practice in a post-transformation period may involve constructing a new "transformed" self that does not deny elements of the previous self that remain.

I experience some degree of detachment from worldly joys and sorrows.

For many people, detachment is a measure of spiritual transformation. Transformation signifies greater present-moment awareness and greater transcendence. From this new vantage point worldly happenings may be seen in a context of expanded time and may seem to occur on a much bigger stage. Commitment to focusing attention on the present—what Eckhart Tolle (1999) calls "the Now"—instead of dwelling on the past or future reduces the potential for a sense of urgency, which is a strong form of attachment. The universal love associated with spiritual transformation enables compassion, a deep empathy with the inevitable discomfort of being human, and humility in the face of trying to do anything about our own and others' suffering. Detachment does not mean that one no longer cares about what is happening to self and others.

I lead a spiritually centered life.

Spirituality shifts from being one among the many self-schemas that form identity to being *a* central or even *the* central schema. Marina's story illustrates this process well.

Marina is in her early 60s and has been on an intentional spiritual journey most of her adult life. She knew at an early age that she was called to a spiritually centered life, and she tried various paths. She entered a convent for a time but found that this life did not suit her. She studied comparative religion, thinking that this might be a way to unite work and spiritual journey. What she found was academic rivalry and discourse that trivialized spiritual experience. Throughout much of her young and middle adulthood, Marina struggled mightily with the whipsaw effects of wanting to conform to the "social program" appropriate to her social class and gender while at the same time trying to lead a spiritually centered life. The empty nest and retirement freed Marina to better integrate her lifestyle and her spiritual life. Her life now revolves around nourishing her inner life and the spiritual lives of others in her spiritual community, as well as serving her community and society by being a quiet but persistent advocate for peace. She is also a mainstay of her spiritual community in terms of willingness to do the instrumental tasks needed to keep the group going.

Marina's lifestyle does not look much like the stereotypical American middle-class picture. She lives in a small but comfortable home, and her love for gardening as a contemplative practice is evident in the well cared-for flower beds surrounding the house. She does not own a television. Marina spends time each day in contemplative prayer, and she also enjoys reading new ideas about various topics concerning spirituality. She teaches classes about different aspects of spirituality, especially the history of mysticism, and takes classes too. She is part of two spiritual discussion groups that meet regularly to share their experiences on the spiritual journey, support one another through difficult times, celebrate life's joys, have fun, and ponder deep questions. Each week, she attends a contemplative gathering of her spiritual community, which has about 125 regular attenders. She also stands at a silent peace vigil each Sunday.

Marina's life looks pretty simple from the outside, but when I listened to all the things she is doing, it brought home vividly Wuthnow's (1998) point that being in charge of one's own spiritual life involves a lot of work. Marina's life is one of deep meaning, incredible joy, the bittersweetness of compassion, strong and enduring relationships, and a persistent tug of work that needs to be done.

I am a spiritual being and not simply a person. I am a spiritual being on a human journey.

Spirituality shifts from being a personal character dimension or focus to being a source of transcendent identity. The personal identity is less important than the transcendent nonpersonal identity. In Hindu philosophy, this is called *realization*, the realization that people have an immortal spiritual aspect that is much deeper than just being a transitory individual. In this philosophy, the supreme being is not an entity but rather an "infinite sea of being." Infinity is difficult to grasp because it is not merely big but is actually limitless—infinitely bigger than big. The Quakers speak of "that of God within everyone." Whatever we conceive God or a supreme being to be, there is a bit of that in us, and we can identify ourselves with it. This idea was also at the root of *The Perennial Philosophy* (Huxley 1944) and Paul Tillich's (1967) idea of a God that served as Ground of God—a God beyond God.

CONCLUSION

There is little question that for many people spirituality is a central element of identity and self. We have looked at a variety of concepts that can be used to detail this relationship. It is also likely that these people navigate the social world in ways that are different from those of people who do not see themselves as spiritual, but much research remains to be done to understand this possibility. My guess is that there is great diversity in the composition of spiritual identity and self and in the ways spiritual identity and self influence lifestyles and life courses. We can also divide those who see themselves as spiritual into those for whom spiritual identity is an ego enhancer and those for whom spiritual identity is a way to transcend ego.

Does our discussion of spirituality, identity, and self imply that incorporating spirituality into identity and self is better than not seeing oneself as spiritual? No. People who see spirituality in their experience are responding to their experience, and people who do not see spirituality in their experiences are also responding to their experience. No implication should be drawn that seeing oneself as spiritual is "better" than not seeing oneself this way. My aim is simply to provide concepts, definitions, and theoretical frameworks that can be used to study spirituality, and these ideas have application mainly for the large proportion of the population who do see spirituality in their world.

This chapter illustrates the difficulty of trying to capture a sense of a person's spiritual identity and self through one-shot survey questions such as "To what extent do you consider yourself a spiritual person?" Narratives of the spiritual journey are particularly informative precisely because they are usually condensed versions of origins, changes, and directions that reflect the underlying values and experiences that shape a specific journey tailored to the needs of a specific person. The many concepts and approaches to looking at spiritual identity and self presented in this chapter are valuable for getting a sense of the important questions to ask, not so much for providing pat answers. They also provide a rich vocabulary that can be used to discuss these important topics.

PART II

Spiritual Journeying

�֍   �֍   ✖   ✖

CHAPTER FOUR

Becoming a Sage and a Spiritual Elder

Transpersonal Psychology

This chapter is about experiences people have in the process of becoming sages and spiritual elders. To become a sage is to manifest wisdom and calm judgment. To become a spiritual elder is to be a sage in the role of elder—in the family, community, or society. A spiritual centeredness is involved in being a sage and in being a spiritual elder. To fully open opportunities for individuals to serve as sages requires a sense that *sage* is a position in the community for which people can be recruited and supported—that sages serve an important function for communities.

I use the word *becoming* to suggest that being a sage is not a destination at which we arrive but, rather, a capacity that we can bring into being in any moment. Becoming a sage in the present moment is the culmination of what has come before in terms of individual spiritual growth and capacity to understand and see clearly the demands of a specific situation. Like a kaleidoscope, the capacity to be a sage is a moving mosaic that requires the ability to be intensely present and at the same time to transcend purely personal perspectives, all the while remaining in touch with a big picture, which moves to bring changing circumstances into focus. Becoming a spiritual elder is also an evolution that couples being and transcendence with action in social roles.

The chapter begins with a consideration of wisdom—what it is and how it develops—because wisdom is the defining capacity of the sage. Next I look at some of the personal, cultural, and social obstacles that prospective spiritual elders must often overcome and the skillful means they might use in manifesting themselves as sages in the community. I then present three types of sage associated with later stages of the life course: sage-in-training, actualized sage, and transcendent sage.

SPIRITUAL DEVELOPMENT AND WISDOM

Like spirituality, wisdom is a sensitizing concept that does not have a concrete referent, so there are many definitions of wisdom. For Paul Baltes and colleagues (Baltes and Smith 1990; Baltes 1993; Baltes and Staudinger 2000), for example, wisdom is merely an advanced form of cognition. In this view, wisdom is a practical skill involving rich factual and procedural knowledge, applied in a context that includes the entire human life course and a multicultural vantage point. As Monika Ardelt (2003) pointed out, this is a Western, instrumental view. For others (Achenbaum 1997; Ardelt 2003; Atchley 1993), an Eastern view, which looks at wisdom as a metaperspective rooted in spiritual development, is necessary if we are to include faculties such as empathy and compassion in the concept of wisdom.

Andrew Achenbaum and Lucinda Orwoll (1991) place growing ability to transcend at the center of their concept of wisdom (see table 8). Their concept of wisdom starts with the spiritual process of transcending at the *intrapersonal* level of the personal self, and this transcendence leads to an expanded, transcendent concept of the self as more than a personal self, a less distorted self-concept, and less self-centered motives for action. When transcendence includes the *interpersonal* level, capacities such as empathy, understanding, and compassion come into play in relationships with others. When transcendence expands to a *universal* level, to include all of life, then self-transcendence is complete and the being recognizes the limits of human knowledge and understanding and is ready to make lasting spiritual commitments. One of Achenbaum and Orwoll's main contributions to the conceptualization of wisdom is including an element of motivation in their definition, the urge to bring spiritual insights to bear on oneself, in one's relationships, and in one's wider world.

TABLE 8
Dimensions of Wisdom: Achenbaum and Orwoll

	Intrapersonal	Interpersonal	Universal
Personality	Self-development	Empathy	Self-transcendence
Cognition	Self-knowledge	Understanding	Recognizing limits of knowledge
Conation	Integrity	Compassion	Philosophical/spiritual commitments

Source: Adapted from Achenbaum and Orwoll (1991).

Ardelt (2003) saw wisdom as an integration of three types of perspective: affective or emotional, cognitive, and reflective or contemplative (see table 9). In the *affective* region, wisdom involves experiences such as compassion, a positive stance toward self and others, and the absence of negative emotions and behavior directed at self or others. In the *cognitive* region, wisdom involves understanding how life works—especially its deeper meaning, human nature, the limits of knowledge, and the fact of uncertainty as part of life. In the *reflective* region, wisdom involves the ability to see what *is* with undistorted perception, to see issues from multiple perspectives, to perceive with less self-centeredness and more self-awareness and insight. To Ardelt, all three of these regions are necessary for fully developed spiritual wisdom.

In the vocabulary we have been using to discuss spirituality, the spiritual qualities of being, transcending the personal self, and direct connection with the sacred are easily integrated into the frameworks developed by Achenbaum and Orwoll (1991) and Ardelt (2003).

Underlying the spiritually focused wisdom frameworks is the notion of a psychology that transcends the personal self and allows for union with the sacred. The term *transpersonal* first came into use to describe an approach to psychology that acknowledges and incorporates the transcendent or spiritual aspects of the human mind that can be joined with cognitive and developmental psychology to create a more holistic approach (Walsh and Vaughn 1993; Wilber 2000). Transpersonal consciousness transcends personal awareness, permitting the experience of a nonpersonal realm within awareness. Transpersonal psychology acknowledges that there are multiple states and levels of consciousness, that psychological development tends toward higher or ultimate human potential, that higher levels of consciousness are nonpersonal or transpersonal in that they are beyond ego-centered consciousness, and that higher levels of consciousness are transcendent and spiritual.

TABLE 9
Dimensions of Wisdom: Ardelt

Affective	Compassion, positive stance toward self and others, absence of negative emotion and behavior toward others
Cognitive	Understanding life's deeper meaning, understanding limits of knowledge and human nature, accepting uncertainty
Reflective	Undistorted vision, multiple perspectives lead to self-awareness, insight, diminished self-centeredness

Source: Adapted from Ardelt (2003).

BEING A SAGE OR A SPIRITUAL ELDER

What does it mean to be a sage? A sage is one who has done the inner work necessary to act in the world with pure being, transcendence of the personal self, and direct connection with the sacred. Sages also manifest cognitive, emotional, and contemplative wisdom. They first must come into deep and enduring contact with their spiritual nature; then they can bring that nature to whatever roles they play in society. In this sense, being a sage modifies how one plays many types of social role, but being a sage is often invisible because it is not based on what we do but who we see ourselves to be as we do it. For every obviously sagely act, the sage performs hundreds of unobtrusively sagely acts. This concept of the sage is flexible enough to accommodate the realities of our postmodern world because it does not center being a sage within a specific role or religious context. However, the spiritual elder can also be a role in itself in contexts that are explicitly spiritual or religious. Spiritual elders are mentors and wisdom keepers, but spiritual elders do not see wisdom as a commodity to possess; they see it is a process that depends on connection to the sacred.

The process of becoming a sage can "transform the downward arc of aging into the upward arc of expanded consciousness" by focusing on the possibility that later life can be a time of unparalleled inner growth (Schachter-Shalomi and Miller 1995, 5–7).

One can be a sage without knowing how to bring this way of being into action. The process of becoming a sage involves an interplay between contemplation and action. Without contemplation, the capacity for action as a sage is not there. For instance, I once attended a meeting at which a venerated Buddhist roshi was present. He sat quietly with great stillness, and at one point the moderator turned to him and said, "Do you have anything to add, Roshi?" The roshi obviously considered the question deeply, and after a long pause said, "No." This no carried much more weight than a casual or offhand no would have. In this case, the action was an obvious act of deeply considering the question and it was rooted in deep contemplation. But without action, there is no sage in the family or community. One may experience enlightenment alone, but for that enlightenment to have effect in the world the enlightened one must continue to participate in the world. When people are recognized as sages—venerated for their experience, judgment, and wisdom and encouraged to play the role of sage—they have become actualized.

OBSTACLES

The cultural concept of life stages and postmodernism constitute important obstacles to becoming a sage. The cultural concept of life stages essentially ignores the potential for spiritual growth, focusing instead on the physical and psychological aspects of maturation and aging, their effects on psycho-biological functioning, and changing social roles. Midlife is seen as being dominated by power and responsibility. Later maturity and old age are seen as life stages permeated by loss, and many people's reaction to this image is denial and avoidance. They avoid aging and older people and deny their own aging. Herein lies another paradox: To become sages, we must embrace all life stages, including later adulthood; but to embrace later life we need positive visions of what it can bring. However, to have positive visions of what later life can bring, we need images of sages. A key to overcoming this obstacle is to recognize that sages are not rare but abundant, if we only know how to look for them.

Postmodernism gives rise to a subjective worldview in which everyone's individual reality is treated as having validity. "My truth" is taken to be each person's ultimate truth. This viewpoint is often used to justify self-indulgence, but it also recognizes a fundamental aspect of human existence: we all have our own personal constructs of goodness, truth, and beauty, which we use to make sense out of life and make decisions about it. This is an important starting point. But instead of taking these personal constructs as ultimate truth, we might consider them as working hypotheses that we are skeptical about, have doubts about, or are willing to subject to the test of dialogue and experience. This last perspective creates experiences of humility in the face of a search for truth. A key is to retain the openness of postmodernism without succumbing to its potential for nihilism.

Fear is probably the major personal obstacle to becoming a sage. We spend many years of our lives learning to function as social beings, and it takes courage to distance ourselves from this type of functioning for a time to learn to function as spiritual beings. Many spiritual seekers find that nourishing spirituality requires a period of intense focus on the spiritual region of experience. A key to letting go of our fear about what may happen to our social functioning as we focus on spiritual development is to recognize that spiritual development does not require that we abandon our lives as social beings. In fact, retaining our capacity as social beings is essential to becoming actualized as a sage. For example, to survive in any social world, one must have a basic understanding of how it functions, including basic ideas about the part we are expected to play. What spiritual development offers is a capacity to see the social world and its demands with more clarity.

We also tend to fear letting go of our social roles. But if we have done our inner work, we can shift our perspective to the spiritual level of consciousness while we continue to function in many of the same social roles. However, we need to have the capacity to remain centered spiritually in order not to be drawn into the materialistic mindset of others we encounter in various everyday venues in which we play our social roles. Many spiritual traditions teach that this learning to be "in the world but not of it" is best begun quietly. Remember, becoming a sage is foremost a way of being and not a set of items on a résumé.

Fear of silence and inactivity is another major obstacle to knowing our spiritual self. In New York, London, or Tokyo, it seems as though most people walking down the street are talking on cell phones. Many people seek to fill every potentially quiet moment with sights and sounds. To those unaccustomed to it, five minutes of silence can seem like an eternity. Those unfamiliar with stillness find it difficult to just sit quietly. Their bodies want to fidget and move. They feel a need to be doing something all the time.

For many people, spiritual development provides an increased capacity to experience silence, stillness, and peace in any moment. One day, as I was rushing to my next meeting, I became aware of how harried I felt. This was a purely "in my head" experience and I was also aware that I was missing out on a beautiful sunny fall day. I shifted my internal focus and began to walk at an amble and to enjoy my surroundings. Instead of arriving at my destination all wound up, I arrived refreshed. Now, I often enjoy the opportunity for stillness and peace that comes with waiting in line. This creates a feeling of the enormity of space and time. In this context, the calm required of a sage is easier to manifest.

Clear seeing also requires that we not turn away from unpleasant truths. Ram Dass (2000, 54) wrote that "in the process of learning to become mindful, and to age in a conscious way, fearlessness is an essential ingredient. This fearlessness involves the willingness to tell the truth, to ourselves and others, and to confront the contents of our minds. We must be willing to look at everything—our own suffering as well as the suffering around us—without averting our gaze, and allow it to *be* in the present moment."

SKILLFUL MEANS

Contemplative practice, spiritual teachings and teachers, and spiritual community are important supports for becoming a sage. Contemplative practices teach us patience. The paradox of contemplative practices is that they are intended to lead us to spiritual experience, yet the harder we try the less likely it is that we will have a spiritual experience. Contemplative practice requires faith because the results of practice are not predictable. By engaging in contemplative practice, we can reduce the clutter in our consciousness and create space within which spiritual experience may occur.

Contemplative practices come in enormous variety, ranging from meditation and contemplative prayer to devotional prayer to rumination on sacred texts to contemplative movement disciplines such as walking meditation and tai chi. All these practices hold the potential to connect us with what Aldous Huxley (1944) and Paul Tillich (1967) termed "the ground of being." The ground of being can be experienced as both immanent and transcendent. It is immanent in that it permeates everything. It is transcendent in that it is experienced as an infinite sea of being. This concept was probably first articulated in Western thought by Meister Eckhart (c. 1260–c. 1327), who said that we need a concept of God as the ground of being against which our more limited personified concept of God can serve as figure. Eckhart Tolle's (1999) concept of the Now is akin to the concept of the ground of being. Countless people have reported that the inner experience of the sacred ground of being is one of deep silence, stillness, well-being, and peace. Once this connection has been experienced, the experiencer is motivated to experience it again. Although contemplative practices cannot guarantee a recreation of the immediate experience of the ground of being, they represent a good strategy. Not only that, but once we get used to the silence and stillness of contemplation, spiritual practice usually becomes a pleasant experience in itself.

Spiritual teachings and teachers can accelerate our spiritual development, but they can also get in the way—yet another paradox. Authentic spiritual teachings about the nature of the spiritually centered life are often attempts to put into words the processes and circumstances associated with an experience of the ground of being. Such teachings come through human vehicles, located in a cultural and historical time and place. Another paradox is that to understand teachings fully, we need to have had our own direct experience of the ground of being. Otherwise the teachings are just thinking. Whether teachings ring true to a person depends on how the teachings resonate with that person's spiritual experiences and the language that seems to him or her to be an authentic way to talk about those experiences. Some people are fortunate to grow up in a spiritual tradition with concepts and language that continue to resonate well with their experiences as they evolve spiritually. Others find that the concepts and language of their religion of origin gradually lose the capacity to describe their spiritual experiences. Often, spiritual seekers remain on the lookout for teachings that express well what they have experienced. It is not that they are necessarily looking for a different truth; they may simply be looking for more or better ways to express what they have already experienced.

Teachers can be invaluable bridges between teachings and experience. Some teachers are good at leading people to a direct experience of the ground of being. Others are good at leading people to ways of expressing those experiences. Some teachers model bringing wisdom into everyday life. Still others are good at many of these things. Not all teachers are gurus. As Ram Dass (1988) said in an audio presentation, "The teacher points the way; the guru *is* the way." Gurus are the embodiment of the teaching in all its aspects. In this respect, the fully realized sage is a guru, although there is no such recognized position in Western societies.

Spiritual communities are a valuable support for the spiritual journey. Some spiritual communities function within the context of traditional religions; others are nondenominational collaborations. Spiritual communities provide guidance, structure, and encouragement. Many people find that being part of a spiritual community makes it easier to sustain their commitment to the spiritual journey. Of course, spiritual communities come in many varieties. Some are loosely organized and democratic in process. Others are hierarchical and doctrinaire. Most are probably somewhere in between these two extremes. Little systematic study has been made of how these variations among spiritual communities influence the nature of spiritual experience or development.

Spiritual communities also serve as a check on the ego's tendency to transform spiritual insights into ego agendas. For example, the Quakers have a process called the "clearness committee," which calls together a small group within the community to help a seeker explore the extent to which a motive is spiritually rooted. Clearness committees are especially likely to be called for those who are considering membership or marriage, but other types of action can also benefit from this process. Clearness committees create a supportive space in which people can, in the company of spiritual peers, explore fully their motives and intentions. Clearness committees are intended not to put a stamp of approval on any particular way of thinking or acting but instead to open an opportunity for the seeker to arrive at greater clarity about the matter.

Being part of a spiritual community also allows a person to explore the language and concepts of spirituality in the company of others who are also confronting issues of spiritually connecting with inner being and transcendence, expressing that connection, and contemplating the implications of that connection for everyday life.

Becoming a sage thus occurs in the context of spiritual development. But it also occurs in a context that includes cultural and personal obstacles both to believing that spiritual growth is the purpose of life and to recovering a role for sages as exemplars of spiritually awakened living. Contemplative practice, spiritual teachings and teachers, and spiritual communities are important supports on the journey to becoming a sage. Becoming a sage is a capacity that usually takes many years to develop.

I have encountered three distinct categories of people who are involved in becoming sages: sages-in-training, actualized sages, and transcendent sages.

SAGES-IN-TRAINING

When a person realizes that becoming a sage is a real possibility, she or he can become a sage-in-training. (Of course, most people who are doing the work to develop spiritual capacities do not see themselves as sages-in-training; that would seem pretentious.) Sages-in-training take on sages as their reference group, people who represent their aspirations. But how do people come to this realization? A fortunate few experience a rite of passage that recognizes their entry into sagehood, but most of us must rely on more subtle messages that we are entering a new stage. Here is my own experience of initiation:

In 1999, I attended an acknowledgment ceremony for elders at Naropa University. The Naropa Elders serve as interview subjects for students, attend classes such as contemplative caregiving or the psychology of aging, and often become mentors for students and faculty. The ceremony was conducted by Subonfu Some, a West African tribal spiritual teacher. In her culture, it is assumed that all elders have done the preparation needed to function as a sage. She began by gathering the elders into a seated circle facing outward. I was surprised when Subonfu took me by the hand and seated me in the circle. Although I was 60, I did not see myself as yet being an elder, and I was easily ten years younger than the others included as elders. There were about fifteen elders in the circle. About seventy-five other attendees (students and faculty) walked around the circle for ten minutes or so singing a lilting song of appreciation to the elders. Then Subonfu instructed the attendees to go to the elders for blessings. I had never in my life given anyone a blessing and had no idea how to do so. A psychology faculty member whom I knew only casually approached me, knelt on the floor in front of my chair, and asked for my blessing. After a brief feeling of being at a loss, I went in my conscious-ness to that place that is beyond my personal concerns and found its stillness. I then lightly placed my hand behind her head and drew her forehead to mine and said, "Be peace." Tears welled in her eyes and she smiled. She then bowed two or three times to me, rose, and stood quietly a moment before moving on. I looked around the room, and the other el-ders were involved in the same unpretentious ritual. I gave different bless-ings to ten or twelve people that day. It seemed that the process of blessing and being blessed was much more important than the specific words. This was my initiation into becoming a sage in the present moment.

Unfortunately, such initiations into sagehood seldom occur in our society. We do not have formal rites of passage that clearly mark entry into elderhood. Instead, if we are lucky we experience subtle messages that people are inter-ested in what we have to offer, especially in situations that involve articulating a big picture. These experiences are openings to practice becoming a sage. Of course, the demands of speaking for the long view, what Ronald Manheimer (1999) called "the work of generations," can also spark an interest in learning more about the role of spiritual elder. But the sagely response in many situa-tions is to sit quietly and wait for a spiritually inspired perspective to appear, and waiting is often not welcome in our fast-paced, multitasking society.

There are a few "schools" where people can learn about being a sage. For example, the Sage-ing Guild is a national network of persons trained to of-fer introductory workshops and several advanced workshops on becoming a sage. The guild workshops support both the inner work that is required to become a sage and the skills and knowledge required to bring that perspective into various roles in the community.

Mentors and role models are also helpful in learning what it means to be a sage. As mentioned earlier, sages are common, but we may need to hone our perception to allow us to see them. In my experience, sages often have notable characteristics in addition to many years of life experience: clarity, patience, an air of quietude, good listening skills, a nurturing attitude toward others, and a lack of anxiety even in the face of distressing circumstances. They may or may not be verbally articulate or interested in social action. By spending time with sages and noticing how they combine their inner work with their capacity to benefit the world, sages-in-training can see that sages come in many varieties and develop a better sense of what it would take to become a sage themselves. Actualized sages are often willing to serve as mentors to sages-in-training.

Inspirational discourse, mentors, and role models are helpful, but the sage-in-training must eventually face alone the inner tasks of spiritual development. These tasks involve cultivating spiritual disciplines, doing philosophical homework, reflecting and integrating, letting go of earlier concerns, practicing forgiveness and gratitude, and making peace with death (Schachter-Shalomi and Miller 1995). These tasks engender a rich inner frame of reference that nurtures the capacity to stay spiritually centered amid the complexities of daily life. They lay the foundation for being able to become a sage in the present moment.

As mentioned, spiritual practices come in many varieties, and to facilitate a steady awareness of spiritual connection with the ground of being, practices are best done regularly. At first, contemplative practices such as prayer or meditation can be difficult. They require being still and quiet as much as possible. The practitioner must learn to push through the urge to abandon practice when the body aches or the mind is filled with cascading thoughts. But the more often the practitioner is able to just sit in awareness of the body and mind, whatever their current state, practice becomes easier. And developing the habit of practice creates a commitment that can carry the practitioner through times when the mind does not want to practice. Developing a mature spiritual practice takes time—years rather than weeks or months.

Practitioners often report feeling that they have gained the ultimate insight only to find that there is more to learn. And much of this learning occurs at an intuitive rather than a verbal or an intellectual level. When this happens over and over again, it instills an attitude of humility, especially because it is so difficult to communicate what one has learned.

What Zalman Schachter-Shalomi and Ronald Miller (1995) call philosophical homework involves contemplating deep questions about where we come from and where we go. They quote Robert de Ropp: "The contemplation of an individual life against the background of time brings inevitably deeper insights into the nature of being and becoming. How vast a time passed before I existed and how vast a time will be after I cease to exist! But what is I? What is this self whose days and adventures are drawing to a close? An isolated spark briefly lit, destined to fade forever into darkness? A fragment of a greater consciousness that will return to the place from which it came? A spirit temporarily imprisoned in flesh? A traveler far from his true home and now about to return?" (124). Who am I? Why am I here? What is my place in the universe? Is there a God? What is God? Can I know God? What is my relation to God? Rumination on these types of questions makes later life a philosophical life stage (Manheimer 1999).

Erik Erikson initially thought that the major psychological task of old age was to develop ego integrity and thus avoid despair in the face of aging and death (Erikson 1955). But in his eighties, Erikson changed his mind. Wisdom was the culminating development of old age, and wisdom was reached by understanding that integrity and despair coexist (Erikson, Erikson, and Kivnick 1986). The wise individual understands that integrity balances despair and that despair tempers integrity. Wisdom thus transcends both integrity and despair. This type of transcendent perspective grows out of years of contemplating deep questions.

To move forward into these deep questions, the sage-in-training must also overcome inertia and let go of earlier concerns. Feeling that one has been wronged or deprived in the past is a major attachment to the past. To move forward, being able to forgive ourselves and those others we hold responsible for past circumstances that distress us is usually helpful. The Buddhist practice of Tonglen (Wegela 1996) is an example of a spiritual practice that can change perceptions of the past and help us develop the compassion that enables forgiveness. The practitioner begins with an attitude of openness, awareness, and compassion. Then he or she focuses for a few moments on the breath, breathing in dark feelings of confusion or pain and breathing out light, bright feelings of relief. Then he or she focuses for a few minutes on a particular situation that causes pain and breathes in those feelings and breathes them back out into the entire universe. Then he or she focuses for a time on all people who experience similar pain, breathing in their pain and then breathing it out into the universe. This last phase leads the practitioner to experience that she or he is not alone in experiencing pain and to experience the relief that accompanies releasing the pain into the vastness of the universe. The result is a feeling of connection and relaxation. From this state, forgiveness and gratitude are much more possible.

Buddhists believe that the reality of death, if unexamined, is like a millstone hanging around the neck. Denying death does not really work. To be free, we must face death and accept it (Becker 1973). To die with awareness, we must be willing to contemplate and ruminate on death until we reach an understanding of it. This is another part of the philosophical homework, dealing with questions such as, How will I deal with the process of dying? What happens to me at the moment of death and after I have died?

Sages-in-training are just getting started on a set of tasks that are rarely fully completed in a lifetime. Just when we think our work is done, life sends us another invitation for further learning.

ACTUALIZED SAGES

Mature adults who have done the inner work that allows them to experience ongoing present-moment awareness and transcendence are able to move about in the world as actualized sages. Generativity and wisdom are the hallmarks of this type of sage.

Generativity involves nurturing and guiding those who will succeed us in the flow of generations (Erikson, Erikson, and Kivnick 1986). It is most often expressed in mentoring relationships. Mentoring is a type of caring relationship; it focuses on accompanying a developing person and providing loving support. Support may involve giving information about a sphere of life, especially an overview, but its ultimate aim is to foster the capacity of the mentee to function on his or her own. Schachter-Shalomi and Miller (1995, 189) assert that "mentors do not impose doctrines and values on their mentees in an attempt to clone themselves. Rather, they evoke the individuality of their apprentices, applauding them as they struggle to clarify their values and discover their authentic life paths." Mentoring is a skill that takes practice, and therefore time, to develop.

Schachter-Shalomi and Miller (1995, 200–202) suggest several guidelines for recognizing the mentoring skills of an actualized sage. First, the sage listens with great spaciousness to the mentee's concerns before attempting to share his or her wisdom. The sage does not expect to transfer great insights unsolicited but instead offers wisdom in small increments in response to questions. Second, the sage uses Socratic questioning methods to evoke the mentee's innate knowing rather than imposing knowledge in an authoritative fashion. Third, the sage does not try to impress the mentee by claiming to be perfect, but instead is an authentic human self—seeking, tentative, and vulnerable. Fourth, the sage works with the mentee's unique human potential, not with some idealization of what everyone should be like. As James Hillman (1999) pointed out, character development is what later life is all about, and character is highly individuated. Fifth, the sage recognizes that the mentoring relationship has phases. In the beginning, there is a gradual development of spiritual intimacy that allows for a genuine relationship. Then there may develop a frequency of interaction that allows the relationship to meet the mentor's need to be of real service and the mentee's need to have someone really understand what she or he is experiencing. The deep trust that this process occasions allows the transmission of wisdom to occur. Finally, the mentee becomes a peer and no longer needs to be under the mentor's wing. The mentoring relationship comes to an end. Both mentor and mentee then need be willing to move forward into a new peer-to-peer relationship.

Mentoring relationships can occur in many different contexts. Parents often mentor their children. Grandparents often mentor their grandchildren. In the workplace, elders can be mentors for those who are at earlier stages in their careers. In community organizations, elders can mentor those who are at an earlier stage of their experience in public service. In almost any intergenerational context, elders can mentor the young. But in our society, too many contexts are age segregated, and the natural tendency of the young to seek mentors among their elders is stifled.

In my course on the psychology of aging, I asked each student to visit an elder who had many years experience on a spiritual path. I had a pool of about thirty such elders who volunteered to be interviewed. Students met with their elder weekly throughout the semester and wrote a ten-page life history of that elder. In the process, more than a quarter of the students became mentees of their elder, and their interactions continued long after the course had ended. Many of these students indicated that had they not been required to meet, they would not have sought out a spiritual elder. In our society, intergenerational contact does not occur naturally, except perhaps in families. Accordingly, for actualized sages to serve as mentors requires that we develop mechanisms to facilitate intergenerational connections. The good news is that intergenerational programming is one of the latest growth areas within gerontology.

As mentioned earlier, wisdom is a quality that sages bring to their own lives and to the social worlds in which they participate. Wisdom is not a commodity that a person can possess. Instead, it is a process that requires skill to enact. In my opinion, the essence of wisdom begins with the capacity to see the world from outside one's own personal agenda. This allows the observer to see various sides of an issue. A person at a transcendent level of consciousness also experiences time in a more expansive way, which creates a more relaxed and less frenzied stance toward decision making. "Being while doing" is a learned capacity that opens opportunities for the quality we call wisdom to enter our world.

To practice bringing wisdom into the world requires developing the habit of being still and patiently awaiting a moment that demands the special gift of nonpersonal perspective that we call wisdom. But, as one sage put it, "In order to bring your special gifts as an elder, you have to be there. You have to resist the temptation to withdraw to the comfort of your own solitude or your small circle of friends. You have to continue to show up in those groups you care about."

Actualized sages, those who are recognized as having the capacity to be a sage in the present moment, generally recognize each other as such and enjoy one another's company. When they get together, there are often periods of comfortable silence. They share their experiences of joy as well as doubt and uncertainty. And there is almost always a sense of the humor that accompanies the human predicament. Rick Moody tells the story of his attending a seminar with the Tibetan Buddhist sage Trungpa Rinpoche in which Moody asked Trungpa, "But doesn't this spiritual practice stuff get boring?" At that point Trungpa took out a water pistol and shot Moody in the face! We have a tendency in our culture to treat spiritual matters seriously, but sages know that there is also great humor in our fumbling attempts to understand the ground of being, connect with that ground, and live from that connection. As Manheimer (1999) pointed out, humor can be an expression of wisdom, the result of a heightened state of consciousness and a philosophical outlook.

Part of wisdom is understanding that we cannot act on every impulse we have to care for others. We have to have as much compassion for ourselves as for those we serve. Actualized sages know that to be able to serve over the long haul requires attention to pacing, establishing a humane life routine. These sages do not try to do everything. They have learned that they must choose wisely how to spend their precious energies.

Actualized sages are "fully operational" but still developing. Moody and Carroll (1997) described a circular process of spiritual growth that begins with a leading, a sense that there is more to be discovered. This creates an opening, during which the spiritual seeker looks around for new opportunities for growth. There is often a struggle as the person attempts to understand and to integrate new understanding with old. Then the individual often breaks through to a new level of integrated understanding. Finally, she or he focuses on how to bring that new insight back into the world. Actualized sages know that they may go through many more cycles of spiritual development. It is a territory that is incompletely mapped, yet actualized sages have faith in the process.

TRANSCENDENT SAGES

Transcendent sages have developed the capacity to abide in the highest levels of spiritual consciousness. They tend to be quiet and to speak only when they have something they feel compelled to say. They are holders of the spiritual field within which others struggle to become and act as sages. They are deeply in touch with a panoramic experience of time.

Ken Wilber (2001) describes the higher levels of consciousness as a "sagely region" that includes a subtle level, which is transindividual and intuitive; a causal level, which is experienced as formless radiance and transcendence; and an ultimate level, in which there is only undifferentiated, infinite consciousness and no separate experiencer. The subtle level of consciousness is the source of the capacities of generativity and wisdom that are the cornerstone of being an actualized spiritual elder.

The causal level of consciousness, which manifests itself as radiance and deep silence and stillness, is the source of the capacity to be a transcendent sage. At this level, there is little that one feels compelled to say, so there is much quietude. Yet there can be great joy in continuing to participate in the routine activities that constitute life, including routine religious and spiritual activities and quiet participation in community.

By abiding at a level of consciousness close to the source of spirit, transcendent sages "hold the field." That is, their presence and quality of being consistently remind more active participants why they are interested in the process of becoming sages. Transcendent sages attract our attention through their manifest connection with the ground of all being. It is not what they *do*, but how they *are* that is their contribution to the group. Consider two examples.

In his mid-80s, William projects an air of robust good health. He attends a worship group regularly, but rarely speaks. Yet he constantly serves as a living example of what it means to be radiantly at peace. He is comfortable with his spiritual nature, and it shows in his clear, soft voice, bright gray eyes, and ready smile. There is a serenity about William's being that many people in the group have remarked on. There is also a sense that the group is missing an important presence when William is not there.

⊕

James attends the same worship group. He is in his early 90s and has numerous chronic conditions that cause him to move about slowly. He is nearly blind and in a great deal of chronic pain. When asked, he acknowledges that his physical existence is not very enjoyable at his stage of frailty. Yet in the worship group, James will occasionally stand and ecstatically recite a psalm from memory. At these times he is completely transported by the Source of the Psalms, and the renderings invariably leave the group uplifted and in awe of this gentle man's connection with God.

Neither William nor James takes a lead in the operation of the group. Focused more on just being present, they leave the logistics to the "youngsters," many of whom are in their 60s and 70s.

Schachter-Shalomi and Miller (1995) assert that sages have a panoramic view of time. Transcendent sages have a type of consciousness that abides "under the aspect of eternity," that sees time not as a commodity or an instrumental need but as a vast panorama, of which our human lifetime is but a small part. Ram Dass (2000, 141) wrote that sages-in-training are learning to live by "soul time" and that souls live by a different calendar, one in which "our egos are like mayflies that are born in the morning and die in the evening." This panoramic view of time redirects values away from the materialistic concerns of our current culture and toward more holistic values, which respect the needs of the entire planet. From a panoramic view of time, we can be patient and persistent and are less likely to become frustrated if we do not immediately achieve our objectives. This perspective on time supports the quietude that characterizes transcendent sages.

Transcendent sages do not stand out. They have little interest in standing out. Yet they are there to see if we only look. Another paradox is that some of the role models we desperately need are right there in front of us, but we don't see them.

CONCLUSION

The idea that elders can possess a high capacity to bring spirituality into their lives and into the world has been around for thousands of years. But what is it about later life that brings this about? The concept of spiritual development presumes that humans have the capacity to evolve spiritually, to identify with their spiritual nature, and, over time, to strengthen their conscious connection to this sacred aspect of self. This development enhances the chances that a person will be able to manifest wisdom as he or she develops spiritually. The concept of the spiritual elder presumes that spiritual development and later life stages can combine to affect how sages act in various social roles and also to prepare individuals to manifest themselves as sages and assume the role of spiritual elder.

Becoming a sage is an evolutionary process through which spiritual development is nurtured, the capacity for wisdom develops, and an individual learns what is needed to prepare for and take up the role of spiritual elder and to be a sage. The openness that aging can create through child launching and retirement can also be an opening to become a sage-in-training. No one knows why some people are drawn to this possibility as a conscious journey, why others unconsciously develop spiritually, and why still others show no signs of spirituality.

Although spiritual development involves continuous cycles of development, being a sage is manifested in ways that are loosely related to stages of later life. At the beginning of later life (the 60s), many people are involved in being sages-in-training, engaging the inner tasks of spiritual growth, and learning from their elders how to behave as a spiritual elder. They are becoming "rooted in their being." In the middle of later life (the 70s and early 80s) many who have been on the journey have become actualized sages, fully in touch with their spiritual nature and able to keep that nature at the center as they function in the world. They are adept at "being while doing." In old age (the mid-80s and older), transcendent sages are common. These people are radiantly at peace and are "being and transcending."

A recurring theme in this chapter has been that sages and spiritual elders are not rare and that by raising consciousness about the characteristics of sages and the process of becoming a sage, we can better recognize them. And as we recognize the extraordinary depth that sages and spiritual elders bring to our collective quality of life, we may come to see value in creating more opportunities for sages to be a more visible part of our world.

CHAPTER FIVE

Transpersonal Sociology and Serving from Spirit

This chapter deals with two questions: How would social organizations look if they were populated, organized, and managed by people with a transpersonal viewpoint and philosophy of life? and, What is spiritually centered service to the community and how does it differ from other kinds of service?

For these questions, the existing literature is of little help. Although organizational management and service are familiar topics in the literature of various religious traditions, in American culture nearly all of this discussion takes a Western, instrumental view of these as practical rather than spiritual concerns. Our literature pays scant attention to the spiritual development of the people in the spiritual community and how it might affect the values of the community, how people are organized to promote those values, the processes spiritually developed people use to approach goals, and how their processes might differ from conventionally organized spiritual communities.

For twenty years I taught organizational management, first for thirteen years in a mainstream academic environment and later for seven years in a university community that aimed to prepare students to approach their work from a contemplative perspective. Because I believe that to teach a subject, one needs experience in the field as well as familiarity with the literature, I did extended field placements and made many site visits to a wide variety of types of organization, particularly professional organizations and service organizations in the field of aging. These experiences provided me with an experiential base I could use to understand how organizations with a critical mass of people with a transpersonal viewpoint differ from organizations that take the hierarchical, competitive approach to organizational life widely used in American culture.

This chapter attempts to present what I have learned about this topic—the ideas I have developed about how organizations and communities can successfully operate using principles of transpersonal sociology. It is necessarily sketchy, and it is filled with conclusions that need to be verified by other investigators. But I think this is an important topic, and I offer this discussion as a starting point, as food for thought, and as a stimulus for future research. In my experience, organizations that operate using principles of transpersonal sociology are much more elder-friendly than are traditional top-down organizations.

WHAT IS TRANSPERSONAL SOCIOLOGY?

The word *trans* is of Latin origin and means beyond, on the other side. The term *transpersonal* first came into use to describe an approach to psychology that acknowledges and incorporates the transcendent, or spiritual, aspects of the human mind, which can be joined with cognitive and developmental psychology to create a more holistic approach (Walsh and Vaughan 1993). Transpersonal consciousness transcends personal awareness and leads to a nonpersonal realm within awareness. Transpersonal psychology acknowledges that there are multiple states and levels of consciousness, that psychological development tends toward higher or ultimate human potential, that higher levels of consciousness are nonpersonal or transpersonal in that they are beyond ego-centered consciousness, and that higher levels of consciousness are transcendent and spiritual.

Transpersonal sociology asks how social psychology, interpersonal relationships, and group dynamics are affected by the presence in a group, organization, community, or society of large proportions of people whose consciousness is at a transpersonal level.[1] In *The Perennial Philosophy*, Aldous Huxley (1944) surveyed the wisdom of sages from a variety of spiritual traditions and wrote that most traditions contain the idea that beyond the phenomenal world of matter and individualized consciousness there is a manifestation in consciousness of what he called "the ground of all being within." The Quakers say, "There is that of God within everyone." The Bible says people are "made in God's image," and this can be taken to mean that God is within us, waiting to be manifested. The Koran says that God pervades everything, including us. Buddhists believe that we all contain a great emptiness or space and that if we dwell in that space, we transcend ego.

Huxley goes on to say that not only can we know the ground of being by intellectual inference, we can also know it directly through contemplative, intuitive methods. So people have a dual nature: a phenomenal ego, which is necessary for survival in the world, and an eternal spiritual self, which is a transpersonal domain and which can be seen as God, the Absolute, the Void, or the Ground of Being. Finally, *The Perennial Philosophy* holds that the primary purpose of life on earth is to identify with and manifest the transpersonal ground of all being.

A MODEL OF TRANSPERSONAL COMMUNITY

Consider what social life would be like if a significant proportion of people in a community lived according to this "perennial philosophy" and had attained the capacity for transpersonal consciousness. How would life be different? That is the subject of transpersonal sociology. Here is how it might look.

Individuals in the community engage in contemplative practices regularly, to nurture their conscious connection with pure being, transcendence, and the ground of being. Children are introduced to contemplative silence early in life by being included in communal silence. Discussions within the community are held against a backdrop of varying degrees of contemplative understanding of the ground of being. Community members know that awareness of the ground of being is "running in the background" of all they do. The experience of inner silence, stillness, and peace seems enhanced by having the experience in a group of people who are all opening themselves to this experience. The group consciously includes periods of silence between topics of discussion to help them remain spiritually grounded. Interpersonal relationships include an element of respect for the ground of being they share. It may not matter whether this is demonstrably true; what may matter is that people in the community act *as if* it were true. This stance toward others nurtures empathy and compassion and respect.

Because all people are assumed to have the potential to transcend the personal and become a voice of wisdom, the community is nonhierarchical, completely democratic, and led by actual consensus. Meetings for decision making contain periodic pauses to remember and silently honor the ground of being that the community wants to be consciously aware of throughout all its discussions. Positions of responsibility are allocated based on individual interest, knowledge, and skills and contain strict term limits to prevent the development of positional power within the community.

In the transpersonal community, the number of years of experience living the culture matter. Elders earn added respect by their way of being, which is honed through many years of practice. Members of the community understand and value the process of "becoming a sage."

Values in a transpersonal community center on nurturing spiritual connection in its people and creating community culture based on that connection. If everyone from all times and all places is assumed to have or have had a spark of the ground of being within themselves, then spiritual texts from a variety of traditions are welcome as food for thought, but authority does not come from texts; it emerges from the collective consciousness of the community, from their contemplative practice together. Members of the community seek to dwell in the now as transcendent beings. As Eckhart Tolle (2003) points out in *Stillness Speaks*, this Now is not a nanosecond but a timeless place, not fixated on ideas of past or future for purposes of manipulation or self-aggrandizement.

Values such as nonviolence, respect, fairness, honesty, integrity, and simplicity are not givens; they emerge out of experience in a transpersonal community. Injunctions to community members tend to be general, and much is left to the contemplative interpretation of the members.

I want to digress briefly to illustrate how this process can lead to a spiritual/ethical framework that can be used to guide community members. In many ways, the Buddhist eightfold path (Surya Das 1997) efficiently describes the general orientation of many groups that use principles of transpersonal sociology.

THE EIGHTFOLD PATH

Wisdom Training
   1. Right View
   2. Right Intention
Ethics Training
   3. Right Speech
   4. Right Action
   5. Right Livelihood
Meditation Training
   6. Right Effort
   7. Right Mindfulness
   8. Right Concentration
(Ibid., 93)

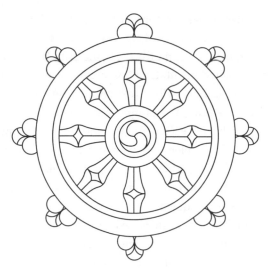

Figure 11. Wheel of the dharma.

The eight subjects contained in the eightfold path are not meant to imply a linear set of steps. Instead, they are depicted as a circle, with all eight topics interconnected at a hub in the middle (figure 11). In the descriptions of the eightfold path, the word *right* is used not in a context of right and wrong but rather in a context of completeness or inclusiveness, coherence, and connectedness.

Thus, right view is facing the ultimate with openness and willingness to transcend the personal. Right intention is aiming to live as much as possible from a nonpersonal, self-transcendent perspective, which supports processes such as good will and nonviolence toward others. Mastering these two topics is called wisdom training.

Right speech involves being aware of the effects of one's speech and using speech in a nonadversarial way. Principles of right speech include: speak the truth—don't lie; use words to help, not harm; don't gossip or tell tales; and speak kindly, not harshly or abusively (ibid., 173–78). Right action involves basic dos and don'ts such as: don't kill; don't take what isn't given freely; give to others in need; refrain from habits that harm body, mind, and spirit. Right livelihood involves making a living ethically and from spiritual consciousness. Together, right speech, right action, and right livelihood are called ethics training because contemplative ethics involves a process of bringing spiritual awareness to these three important areas of life.

Right effort involves a passion for spiritual growth. Right mindfulness involves being rooted in the Now, and right concentration involves being able to remain focused spiritually amid the trials and tribulations of everyday life. These capacities are called meditation training because they deal with different aspects of remaining spiritually awake and paying attention.

The eightfold path is but one example of a system designed to give guidance to those who wish to live a spiritually centered life. Its main virtue is its generality. How each of the elements plays out in an individual life depends on how that individual engages life issues with mindfulness and transpersonal awareness. Group culture built up from this process is different from group culture that is imposed "top down."

Now let us return to our example community. Within the community, small groups of members gather to gently serve others who are struggling with their spiritual journey, mostly by compassionate listening. The contemplative group process in the community minimizes the possibility that the group will be led astray by a charismatic egotist, because decisions are not made in haste and must be based in consensus. By the time everyone is persuaded of the value of a course of action, it is unlikely to be based in someone's misguided or self-centered interpretation of a situation. This does not mean that decision making is easy, and often a clear course of action may take some time to appear. Mistakes happen and so does self-forgiveness, both within individuals and within the community.

Clearness is a vital part of the process. When people regularly practice coming to discussion from a place of contemplation, transpersonal consciousness, and beingness, their capacity to see the world as it is and not as they might wish it to be is greatly enhanced. Compassion is a second vital element. Compassion is rooted in universal love, an experience that does not come through personal consciousness but through transpersonal or nonpersonal consciousness. Compassion is not the overly idealistic romantic love that we see in movies or on television. It is a feeling of enormous well-being that comes with the experience of being connected to all things through the ground of being.

Parker Palmer (2004) tells the following story, which he calls "true community."

> Five years after leaving Berkeley, I found myself sitting in circles again. This time it was at Pendle Hill, a Quaker living-learning community near Philadelphia, where I spent eleven years starting in the mid-1970s. But these

circles, I soon discovered, were of a different sort. They were not heady, aggressive, self-congratulatory, or manipulative. They were gentle, respectful, and reverent in the way they honored self and world, and slowly they changed my life.

In these quiet Quaker circles, people were doing neither the amateur psychotherapy nor the faux politics that I had experienced in Berkeley. Instead, they were doing therapy and politics rightly understood: reaching in toward their own wholeness, reaching out toward the world's needs, and trying to live their lives at the intersection of the two.

In these quiet Quaker circles, I saw people challenged, but I never saw anyone harmed. I witnessed more personal transformation than I had seen before, and I watched more people embrace their social responsibilities as well. That was when I started to understand why Quakers, who have always been few in number, have often been over-represented in the great social issues of their time.

The circles of trust I experienced at Pendle Hill are a rare form of community—one that supports rather than supplants the individual quest for integrity—that is rooted in two basic beliefs. First, we all have an inner teacher whose guidance is more reliable than anything we can get from a doctrine, ideology, collective belief system, institution, or leader. Second, we all need other people to invite, amplify, and help us discern the inner teacher's voice for at least three reasons:

The journey toward inner truth is too taxing to be made solo: lacking support, the solitary traveler soon becomes weary or fearful and is likely to quit the road.

The path is too deeply hidden to be traveled without company: finding our way involves clues that are subtle and sometimes misleading, requiring the kind of discernment that can happen only in dialogue.

The destination is too daunting to be achieved alone: we need community to find the courage to venture into the alien land to which the inner teacher may call us.

I want to dwell for a moment on that little word discern, which means "distinguishing between things." I think again of C. S. Lewis's tales of Narnia, that land of inwardness the children enter through the back of the magical wardrobe. There is much in Narnia that is good and beautiful, especially the voice of truth—the voice of Aslan, the great lion—that is sometimes heard in the land. But there are other voices in Narnia as well, voices of temptation, deception, darkness, and evil. It takes four children, a variety of guides, and seven volumes of pitfalls and perils to sift through this mix of messages and travel toward the truth.

Occasionally, I hear people say, "The world is such a confusing place that I can find clarity only by going within." Well I, for one, find it at least as confusing "in here" as it is "out there"—usually more so!—and I think most people do. If we get lost in New York City, we can buy a map, ask a local, or find a cabbie who knows the way. The only guidance we can get on the inner journey comes through relationships in which others help us discern our feelings.

But the kind of community I learned about at Pendle Hill does not presume to do that discernment for us, as communities sometimes do: "You tell us your version of truth, and we will tell you whether you are right or wrong!" Instead, a circle of trust holds us in a space where we can make our own discernments, in our own way and time, in the encouraging and challenging presence of other people. (25–27)

Although most spiritual communities operate using conventional ideas about authority structures, hierarchical power structures, and bureaucratic rational-legal organizing principles, there are spiritual communities that have for centuries been trying to live by principles of transpersonal sociology.[2] Much can be learned from them about transpersonal sociology.[3]

A major benefit I have observed in the transpersonal approach to community is the large extent to which such organizations avoid the problem of alienation. When everyone is part of every solution, there are fewer divisive problems. When "the power structure" is all of us, against whom could we revolt? This is not to say that there is no sense of discomfort or dissatisfaction; these seem to be human inevitabilities. But direct democracy, consensus decision making, centering on sacred silence, and limits on personal power are principles that could be widely applied, and in this context dissatisfaction is more often met with caring concern rather than impatience or anger. Clearness and compassion are the roots of authentic, unselfish service. Clearness allows us to see what is needed, and compassion creates the capacity to face our own suffering and that of others. Serving in a context of spiritual community is a highly effective mode. Now let us look further at how transpersonal sociology might be actualized through serving from spirit.

SERVING FROM SPIRIT

This discussion is intended as a guide to understanding and practicing spiritually centered service. It is both speculative and utopian. The subject would be an excellent topic for research, especially because the major public effort to encourage increased service by elders, Civic Ventures, says nothing explicitly about spirituality and its relation to service. My thesis is that much service is motivated by the fact that for many people, service is a spiritual experience. For many people, service is a source of much joy and satisfaction. *Uplifting* is a word often used to describe experiences of service.

The serving-from-spirit concept is based on the idea that effective service in the community is rooted in two things: a cultivated connection with the experiential spirituality that lies within each human being, and knowledge and skills needed to be effective in whatever arena of service one chooses. Serving from spirit is a stance from which to be of service and a model of how one can grow spiritually while becoming more effective in service to the community.

In *How Can I Help?* Ram Dass and Paul Gorman (1985) assert that service stems from the human impulse to care. We can see this especially clearly in how communities respond to disasters such as floods or tornados. At such times, the impulse to care for one another is overwhelming. The impulse to care is a noble inclination, but it tells us little about how to care or what will be effective. Service over the long run requires that we build on the impulse to care.

The serving-from-spirit model begins with the goal of being spiritually grounded while serving. As people grow spiritually, they develop levels of consciousness and awareness that alert them to the obstacles thrown in their paths by our self-centeredness. Ego-based service is first and foremost about the ego's needs. A reflective process of examining personal motives for serving can help identify ego-based motives. Enlightened service rises above the ego to more clearly see what is needed. To move toward enlightened service requires skill in remaining spiritually centered while doing the work of service.

Many well-intentioned people find their service less satisfying than they would like because they do not have essential information about the structure and operation of the field in which they wish to serve. Most areas of service have their own unique concepts and language about what they do and how they do it. "Paying your dues" involves getting the experience needed to ensure being sufficiently informed to serve effectively. This does not mean passively accepting other people's definitions of what is good, true, or beautiful; it means making sure to understand the situation before weighing in with suggestions for change.

A person who is accomplished at serving from spirit is able to stay spiritually centered amid the ups and downs of working in an organizational environment, often in situations involving people who are in desperate need. Those serving from spirit are also knowledgeable about how to work within the organizational context and with the types of people who are to be served.

LISTENING TO ONE'S ENTIRE BEING

People find their way to spiritual paths and to community service in many ways. The mind, the ego, the heart, the body, and the soul can each lead us. But if people are only listening to one part of being, then they are not taking advantage of all their resources for being clear about what they are doing or thinking about doing. Listening to one's entire being involves cultivating sensitivity to each dimension of being. This possibility is greatly enhanced by contemplative practice—meditation, rumination, and inner stillness and quietude. In this sense, contemplative practice is an important companion on both the inner spiritual journey and the outer journey of service. Contemplative practice can put people in touch with higher levels of consciousness, from which it is possible to see clearly the workings of mind and ego, true compassion, actions that would truly be of service, and a pace that is healthy for the body.

MINDFULNESS AND TRANSCENDENCE

Mindfulness and transcendence are important qualities to bring to the spiritual journey and to bring to service. Mindfulness is being right here, right now. It is an intense awareness of the present moment. With mindfulness people are able to see more clearly what is before them. They are more likely to see what will actually be helpful in serving another human being or serving an organization. In this framework, it is not so much a matter of doing for others as *I* would like to be done for, but doing for others as *they* would like. It is a matter of doing service that is not self-centered.

To employ mindful service, we also need a vantage point that transcends our ordinary consciousness of self. Ordinary consciousness is ego-centered.

We are the main character in the drama. But as soon as we begin to witness our ordinary self, we have transcended that self and can see it more clearly than we possibly could from the middle of our ego-agendas of desire or fear. To the witness, we are only one of the characters in the drama and not necessarily the most important one at a given moment. When we look into the eyes of another person and realize that we are looking at another being just like us, we can experience a unity-level of consciousness. Witness and unity consciousness are both transcendent levels of awareness that make it more possible to grow spiritually and to serve effectively.

BECOMING WISDOM AND COMPASSION IN ACTION

Being wise and having compassion are not all-or-nothing conditions. They are qualities that exist in degrees. They are not something we have but are capacities we can develop. They are qualities that we *might* be able to bring into being in a given situation. If we have cultivated wisdom and compassion, we have a greater capacity to manifest those qualities, but this happens in the present moment. Whether we can manifest wisdom and compassion depends on how centered we can remain. When we are in a situation of service, we are usually called to be wise and to be compassionate. How well we can do this depends a great deal on how long we have been practicing wisdom and compassion. In practice, a circle of sages is always more effective than a single sage precisely because even sages cannot be all things to all people.

Often we think of service as something that involves volunteering or working within an organizational context. However, service is really an intention that we can take with us into a wide variety of situations. What would happen if we went joyfully about our daily lives seeing every person as someone we could potentially serve, in however small a way? What would happen if we took every opportunity to tend our planet and our environment? Often these do not involve big programs or long-term tasks but are things we can do moment by moment by moment. It takes only a few minutes to listen intently to someone who needs a receptive ear; it takes only a few seconds to pick up a piece of trash. The feeling of service is something that happens in the present moment, whether we are doing it in an organizational context or on our own.

OBSTACLES TO EFFECTIVE SERVICE

Ego often blinds us to what is needed. We sometimes focus on our needs rather than the needs of those being served. In service, the Golden Rule is not serving as *we* would want to be served but instead serving others as *they* want to be served. It is difficult to provide client-centered service from the point of view of our own personal ego agenda.

Lack of background in the field in which we wish to serve can waste time and energy because we don't realize what we don't know and spend time re-inventing the wheel. By patiently and humbly assisting and working alongside skilled people who are already familiar with the service environment and its demands, we can efficiently gain the knowledge and skills we need.

Lack of clarity can result when we are too close to a situation. To achieve a clearer vision of what is needed, we need to have a bigger picture. We can then see ourselves, other servers, those being served, and the context for all of it at the same time.

Professional standards of service are helpful when they convey practical knowledge or guidelines that improve service. However, when professional standards are used to create monopolies of opportunity to serve, they get in the way of the expression of the impulse to care.

We all have a threshold of sacrifice, a level of contribution of time and money that we can devote to service and still be able to meet other important obligations to ourselves, our family, and our community. When we pass this threshold for a lengthy period, we can find ourselves in conflict that reduces our capacity for effective service.

PAYING ONE'S DUES

Each new service environment we enter has its own language and customs, and we need to give ourselves time to assimilate these elements. Otherwise we risk behaving in ways that seem arrogant, naïve, or clueless to those already working in the environment. Curiosity and humility provide a useful stance from which to pay one's dues and earn the respect of others in the environment. It is helpful to be careful about assuming that knowledge from another field can be readily adapted to a new situation. Asking lots of questions and asking for help learning the ropes can be useful strategies.

Much of our service occurs in an organizational context. What are the mission and vision of the organization? What values serve to anchor its operation? What are its major goals? What outcomes does it seek? To what extent are the clients involved in setting goals? Who are the major stakeholders in the success of the organization? These and many other questions create a big picture within which our service work will take place. It's important to know how our work fits into the whole.

TAKING CARE OF ONESELF

Effective service is based in a balance between caring for others and caring for oneself. Each of us needs rest, nourishment, and perspective if we are to be able to serve over the long run. Rest is not just sleep, although sleep is important. Rest also occurs when we pace ourselves so that we are not living in a perpetually rushed state. Nourishment of the body is equally important, but so is nourishment of the mind and spirit. Contemplative reading of sacred texts or books and articles on spiritual themes is an example of a practice that nourishes the mind. Meditation is an example of a restful practice that nourishes the spirit. Movement disciplines such as yoga and tai chi can stretch and relax the body and release built-up tensions. Leading a contemplative life aimed at nurturing the whole person provides a perspective that allows us to bring enough love to our acts of service that we can endure the pain of compassion.

DOES LIFE STAGE MATTER?

If we think about stages of adulthood in terms of issues and challenges of young adulthood, middle age, later adulthood, and old age, then there are major differences in terms of competition from interests other than community service, effects of the amount and type of life experience, and interest in an intentional spiritual journey.

In young adulthood, people often focus on finding a livelihood that is right for them and making decisions about mate selection and family formation. By the time people reach middle age, their job and family responsibilities often become routine, perhaps still demanding but well within their capacity, and opportunities for community involvement often increase. In later adulthood, having launched children into adulthood and having retired from the workforce can bring increased freedom to choose a life of community service. In old age, many people maintain their involvement in community organizations, especially religious organizations, and a few find themselves serving as sages or spiritual elders.

In terms of the intersection of spirituality and community service, young adults often experience strong pressures to concentrate on employment and family, both of which can mobilize the impulse to care. For many young adults, issues concerning the meaning of life have not yet stimulated them to think about a conscious spiritual journey. By the end of young adulthood, most people have had enough experience living with the results of their own actions to have deep respect for the difficulties of deciding the right course of action.

By middle age, many adults have begun to question materialistic culture's definitions of the good life. Many have followed society's prescription for life satisfaction only to find the results less than satisfying. They may then embark on a search for meaning, and the world's wisdom traditions offer many spiritual paths for finding it. At the same time, increased opportunities for community involvement and service can provide an experience of meaning through service. The spiritual journey and the journey of service can complement each other.

Later adulthood can also bring a need for new direction. Those who did not develop an orientation to serving from spirit in midlife may find themselves drawn to it later, as child launching and retirement create opportunities to rethink one's lifestyle. After a period of resting up from the demands of middle age, many people at the beginning of later adulthood begin a period of experimenting with various ways to lead a satisfying life. Eventually, some settle into a life focused on community service.

In old age, there are adults who are uniquely qualified to serve as sages and spiritual elders—individuals who combine a deep spiritual connection, insights based in their considerable life experience, and concern for nurturing the upcoming generations of adults. As parents, many spiritual elders help ease the transition of their offspring into later adulthood. They serve as role models and mentors for middle-aged and older adults as well as for young people. Spiritual elders continue to participate in the life of the community, but they have often moved beyond the need to take an operational leadership role.

CONCLUSION

In this chapter I have looked at how groups, organization, communities, and society might be affected by the presence of a large percentage of people with a transpersonal perspective. I have also looked at how spirituality might influence aging in community. I began with a description of the "perennial philosophy" as a way of understanding spirituality that might apply across many religious cultures. I then used this philosophy to describe how a community might work if it were committed to making spirituality a full partner with other aspects of community culture. I also considered how service might look if it were motivated by a transpersonal perspective. The description of transpersonal community may seem utopian, but communities all over the world are attempting to live this way. They offer much food for thought about the possibilities for aging in such communities.

As plausible as the material in this chapter might appear, or not, the research behind it consists mostly of my own observations of aging individuals and a limited number of organizations and communities over the past fifteen years. The ideas here are best looked at as a complex of concepts and hypotheses that might guide further study in this area.

PART III

Examples Using an Expanded View

✥   ✥   ✥   ✥

✢ ✢ ✢ ✢

CHAPTER SIX

Continuity, Spiritual Growth, and Coping in Later Adulthood

Despite a social world that has a negative orientation toward aging, most aging and older people have good health, high self-acceptance and self-esteem, a high degree of life satisfaction, a satisfying and meaningful lifestyle, and a long-standing convoy of social support (Atchley and Barusch 2004). This happens because over decades of life experience, a large majority of adults have developed robust ideas about what they want out of life and how to get it. Most people don't just sit back and let life happen; they try to influence the directions it takes for them. They usually understand that they don't control life's direction, but they believe they can influence it. They have enduring values that serve as the basis for their life structure, their day-to-day decision making, and their vision of a desired future. They are also resilient; they have encountered enough surprises, contradictions, and paradoxes in life to know that they have to pay attention and cope when the situation demands it. What they have learned from life is a powerful resource for coping. Most have also discovered that coping is easier when done with the support of others.

Focus on the inner life, service to others, and deepening connection with the sacred are bright spots of growth and development for most elders. Many elders see these trends as fully available to them and as goals around which they can organize their lives. The sense of optimism and equanimity that comes from leading this sort of life is also a great resource for coping.

When we see elders for whom things have gone awry, we can look to their personal systems for clues concerning unwanted discontinuities, an inadequate sense of meaning, and a murky view of where they are headed.

Thus, the strong coping capacity most elders possess rests on an equanimity that comes from continuity of values, lifestyles, and relationships, plus turning to spirituality as a frontier of individual development and community formation. Continuity provides a benchmark for organizing thoughts and action; spiritual development provides a spacious context and an expansive perspective, which can foster a sense of equanimity even in the face of adversity.

I will explore each of these topics in more detail. Data to support the various ideas presented come from my twenty-year longitudinal study of aging and adaptation (Atchley 1999) and from my research on spiritual development and service in later adulthood (Atchley 2000, 2003, 2005).

CONTINUITY

Continuity is dynamic and evolutionary. Like continuity in a stage play, continuity here means a character evolving over a lifetime of action and learning and struggle and joy and heartbreak. The character remains recognizable in most cases, but evolution is also obvious. Continuity of personal style, values and beliefs, lifestyles, and relationships constitutes a solid base from which to greet changes in circumstances, both positive and negative.

Using the results from a longitudinal study that began with 1300 people age 50 or older in 1975, whom I followed for twenty years, I was able to look at internal continuity of ideas and external continuity of activities and relationships as respondents adapted to aging. Details of this study were published in Atchley (1999). Here are some of the major conclusions:

— Continuity means evolutionary consistency and linkage over time; stability or equilibrium is a type of continuity, but evolutionary forms of continuity are more common.

— Continuity over time is often seen in the psychological, behavioral, and social patterns of aging individuals. As a theme, continuity is highly integrated with many aspects of life.

— Continuity usually coexists with discontinuity, and continuity far outweighs discontinuity.

— Continuity is more evident in general patterns than in the specifics subsumed thereunder.

— Individual perceptions of reality consist of personal constructs that individuals actively develop by learning from life experience.

— Individual patterns of adaptive thought continue to develop throughout life.

— Using continuity strategies to pursue goals and adapt to change does not necessarily lead to successful results, but if we take life satisfaction as a measure of success, then continuity is usually a successful adaptive strategy.

— General patterns of thought, behavior, and relationships are robust and can accommodate considerable change in detailed patterns without triggering a sense of discontinuity.

— Through decision making about self-concept, life course, and lifestyle and experiencing the consequences, individuals acquire a sense of personal agency and efficacy.

— Enduring patterns of thought, behavior, and relationship are the result of selective investments of time and attention made by individuals over a period of many years.

— Continuity of general patterns of thought, behavior, and relationship is the first strategy people usually attempt to use to achieve their goals and adapt to changing circumstances.

— Continuity of personal goals provides people with an enduring sense of developmental direction.

(Adapted from Atchley, 1999: 151–54)

In general, findings from both qualitative and quantitative analyses of the longitudinal study data strongly supported these conclusions. The findings support the idea that continuity is multidimensional. Continuity does not occur by inertia or chance; it was recognized as an intentional choice by a large proportion of the respondents.

Most people develop a personal system that is a result of decades of learning through life experience. Some people don't learn much from life, but most do. Their personal system is a reflection of their values and their experiences trying to live by them. Values are some of the most enduring inner constructs we have. They fuel our aspirations and our fears.

By late middle age, most adults have developed self-confidence, a feeling that they can influence their own fate. In fact, only about 1 percent of the participants in my longitudinal study had low self-confidence. Most also had a high degree of emotional resilience. Health was the factor most likely to affect both self-confidence and emotional resilience, but even people who had poor health and functional disability seldom had low self-confidence or lacked emotional resilience.

"Being able to accept myself as I am" was a prevalent personal goal, which became stronger over time. This reflects a shift in orientation from self-esteem based on feedback from others to self-esteem based on an inner integration, which Erikson, Erikson, and Kivnick (1986) referred to as integrity.[1] Other important self-referential values included being dependable and reliable and being self-reliant. People wanted to be able to be counted on and to stand on their own two feet. They wanted to be seen as a good person by others. The resilience of these values even in the face of substantial disability suggests that as long as people saw these values at work in their lives in some fashion, self-respect could be maintained. And this self-respect was rooted in realism, not idealism.

In later adulthood, respondents also valued social connections with family and friends, with family having primacy for most people. More than 80 percent felt that it was important to have at least one close, intimate relationship. Having a confidant was important for both men and women. By late adulthood, values such as being prominent in the community or being accepted by influential people were unimportant for most respondents. I found a high prevalence of continuity over time in values, with 80 percent of study participants showing evolution within a basic value framework over the twenty-year period.

Lifestyles are constructed to produce life satisfaction, and life experience tells us how well we are doing with that. By later life, most respondents had settled into a lifestyle that reflected their values and that was robust in terms of helping them adapt to change.

Over the twenty years of my longitudinal study, continuity of activities occurred most commonly for reading (83.5%), being with friends (75.4%), being with family (67.5%), attending church (66.9%), and gardening (56.6%). Note that most of these activities are ones that an individual can easily adapt to changes in health. In overall activity patterns, few study participants took up new activity areas as they aged. Most adjusted their level of participation in activities with which they already had experience. When I looked at how respondents adapted to functional losses, most were able to maintain the same pattern of activity at a lower level of participation. This allowed them to continue to get satisfaction from the same lifestyle despite functional limitations or changes in living arrangements.

Life experience is filled with paradoxes, contradictions, and ambiguities. Relationships, especially the convoy of social support, help us understand the nuances of life, grapple with decision making under conditions of uncertainty, and receive comfort in times of trial.

SPIRITUAL DEVELOPMENT

Spiritual development supplies new perspectives and motives that provide a renewed sense of direction in later life. It is promoted by questions such as, Is this all there is? What does it all mean? How do I fit into the picture? What will happen to me when I die? How can I leave a legacy for future generations? How can I give back to a world that has nurtured me? Do I need to get even with a world that hasn't nurtured me? These and many other questions fuel a spiritual journey that for most people becomes more intentional in midlife. This happens as parents begin to age and experience frailty, as family and cohorts begin to die in larger numbers. It can also result from having been successful and finding that success doesn't provide the meaning we were led to expect.

At its heart, the spiritual journey is about becoming rooted in being, about nurturing and living in a connection with the ground of being, however labeled. It is also about developing a perspective about life that transcends the purely self-centered. Nonpersonal consciousness combines with spiritual development to create a channel for the universal love that is compassion. Compassion is a prerequisite for meaningful service. It takes a lot of compassion to be with others' suffering.

> Within each I Am lies the great source of all being
> Light from within, that's our illumination
> To dwell in silent peace and stillness, that's our meditation
> To see the passing world with clearness and compassion
> And when we clearly see, we are drawn to BE love and to serve.
>   (Adapted from Atchley, 1996)

Many elders participate in small circles of friends who support one another on their life journeys, including their spiritual journeys. There are also groups that focus their attention specifically on the spiritual journey. Many religious communities have numerous small groups that serve this purpose. They may be called study groups, women's groups, men's groups, or issue groups, but many of them also provide support to the group members as they grapple with life issues, including spiritual development.

Not everyone is lucky enough to be part of a spiritual community that fosters such groups. The Sage-ing Guild was created both to promote inner spiritual work and to recover the role of sage in the community. It offers educational programs and resource materials, especially concerning how to form, facilitate, or convene small groups aimed at spiritual development and spiritually centered service (see www.sage-ingguild.org). The point here is that spiritual development often occurs spontaneously and naturally, but because it is an enjoyable purpose we may also be attracted to a conscious spiritual journey, either alone, in the company of others, or both.

Spiritual development is in essence an increasing connection with the nonpersonal ground of being that lies within each human being, whether he or she is religious or not. Spiritual development leads people toward deeper spiritual experience, an expansive view of time and space, and the joy of service for its own sake. For those drawn to it, spiritual experience gradually infuses more and more of life, until most experiences are at least partly a spiritual experience.

Because joy in the act of serving comes to be its own reward and doesn't depend on social acknowledgment, it is available all the time. Spiritual development creates an increasingly large space in consciousness, and in that large nonpersonal space, it is possible to see the ups and downs of the world with something approaching compassion and equanimity.

Most elders continue to serve their families, but in new ways that tap into the wisdom that comes with learning from a lifetime of experience. For most people, the role of grandparent is a wonderful mix of caring and mentoring, without the heavy childrearing responsibilities of parenthood. It is one of later life's greatest service opportunities, and in it, we serve not only our grandchildren but our children as well.

Most elders gradually learn compassionate listening, which creates space for younger people to express their hopes and fears and often opens the door for mentoring, which is in many ways the social equivalent of being a midwife. The mentor doesn't determine the nature of the new being, just eases the birth.

Most elders are part of circles of friends who support one another by providing a safe context for learning and coping. Often, elders are also very much in touch with nature's need for us to serve it. Caring for plants, animals, and the natural environment seems an important way to be rooted in the earth.

Years of being on a path of service leads to an understanding that every contact with every thing can be an opportunity for service, so we don't have to worry about opportunities. We may have long-term service commitments we are willing to make, but we also are awake to opportunities that spontaneously arise to be helpful. To know what is needed, we must clearly see, which is very much a spiritual practice. Clear seeing demands that we be able to stand outside our personal agendas, and spiritual development promotes this process.

When we are committed to service, we see opportunities everywhere and we don't have to be preoccupied with whether we have the "authority" or are "required" to serve.

COPING

In combination, continuity and spiritual development explain why a large proportion of elders adapt well to the ups and downs of aging. But let us look more closely at the dynamics of coping.

Continuity is an adaptation strategy. When people need to adapt, more than 90 percent first try solutions that have worked for them in the past, use self-knowledge to make decisions, and lean toward activities that have already proved satisfying. Nearly 90 percent have a personal philosophy of life that is a consistent force in the decisions they make.

In terms of specific patterns, how people adapt is highly individualized. But we can make a few general statements based on my twenty-year study (Atchley 1999). First, relationships are a vital element of adaptation for most people. When asked, "What enables you to cope? What keeps you going?" most people speak first of family and friends. Having a positive attitude is a close second. This is expressed in many ways: a sense of humor, looking on the bright side, being determined or strong, loving life, enjoying little things. Such an attitude is highly related to level of self-confidence. Religiousness and keeping busy are a distant third and fourth. Some people mention immersion in nature as a way to put their troubles in perspective.

Spiritual development is one of the few goals that increase in importance with age. In my longitudinal study, for example, at the last data point (1995), everyone was age 70 or older. Seventy-nine percent said that their inner life was more important to them then than when they were 50 (Atchley 1999). Spiritual development supports adaptation by fostering a perspective in which time becomes panoramic and space become infinite. In such a context, there is less to be anxious about.

As mentioned earlier, Lars Tornstam's (2005) theory of gerotranscendence holds that as people age they gradually transcend the biological, psychological, and social bonds that cause us all so much anxiety. In my longitudinal study, I found that, compared with when they were 50, a large proportion of respondents said that they were less afraid of death now, felt a greater connection with the universe, and got more enjoyment from their inner life (Atchley 1999).

When we see elders just sitting, we are quick to assume that there is nothing going on, but we may be wrong. I had the following conversation with an 80-year-old woman:

> "There are times when you seem to be in a far-off place in your mind," I said.
>
> "Yes," she said.
>
> "Is it a pleasant place?" I asked.
>
> "Oh, my, yes," she said.
>
> "Can you tell me what it is like?" I asked.
>
> She replied, "Words don't describe it. It's warm and cozy. Thoughts come and go, but are of no importance. I feel completely at peace."

No wonder she liked to have her contemplative time in the afternoons.

We should be careful not to assume that everyone needs to be busy all the time. Contemplative time is important, too.

SPIRITUAL NEEDS

Elizabeth MacKinlay (2006, 69) wrote that "if we do not assess for spiritual needs, we will not even begin to notice these needs nor begin to find ways of addressing them. As I see it, spiritual needs underlie the psychosocial needs of people—they lie at the very core of what it is to be human. If we neglect these, especially for people at critical points of their lives and for those who are facing their frailty, dying, and death, then we neglect something equally important as failing to provide food. . . . Spiritual care can no longer be an optional care component." MacKinlay sees the need for meaning as the most fundamental spiritual need. Creating a spiritual life that provides a sense of ultimate meaning gives a resource for putting life events, both positive and negative, into context, transcending losses and disabilities, creating a sustaining sense of connection with the sacred, and developing the capacity for deep inner peace.

Because spirituality is highly subjective, assessing spiritual needs does not lend itself to standardized approaches to needs assessment. While writing this book, I talked with many people about their spiritual journeys, and in these conversations I was struck by how often the spiritual process involved contemplating and working with profound questions. I began writing these questions down and organizing them into categories. Then I began offering them to people as a resource for personal spiritual self-assessment. Many people found them useful, and many also found them daunting. These questions are reproduced in this book as Appendix B, Questions for Reflection and Spiritual Self-Assessment. The format supports self-assessment, but the questions could easily be modified for use as a way of finding out about spiritual needs. Spiritual needs, which are not apparent on the surface, are some of the most subjective, deeply private needs we have, and approaching them through asking general questions has worked well for me. In interviews, I also found it best to begin with one or two basic questions rather than overwhelm the respondent with the full list.

CHALLENGES TO COPING

Most elders live in a world in which continuity and spiritual development are robust resources for coping. However, two things can happen to make elders more vulnerable: disability and thinning of the social network. When this happens, continuity needs to be seen as evolutionary, not business as usual. With brittle continuity, elders try to maintain independence, often at the expense of social contact. Elders needing long-term care prefer to get it at home, but unless they have a rich social network indeed, they may find themselves increasingly isolated.

Research shows that elders are constantly making new acquaintances and developing new friendships. But as people become homebound, this becomes more difficult. Unless they are tied into a community with strong outreach, elders can find themselves in a situation in which the only people they see are those who are paid to visit—often not a good situation. Mrs. E's story illustrates the difficulties increased disability can pose for those who "age in place."

> Mrs. E lived in a small city of 25,000 in the Midwestern United States. At 65, she lived alone, but was active in her community. She founded a singles group for middle-aged and older adults and was active in state politics, often hosting visiting candidates and doing logistics for their events. She spent her time caring for her small home, flower arranging, and visiting with her many friends. She was also close to two older sisters who lived about an hour's drive away. Her life was full of activity, she found meaning in relationships, and she also enjoyed her solitude.

At 75, Mrs. E had had a stroke, which left her balance impaired and required that she give up driving and use a three-wheeled walker to get around. Gradually she lost contact with many of her friends. They came to see her at first, but as the months went by they gradually stopped visiting. Her sisters were also becoming more impaired, and their visits became much less frequent, although they kept in touch by phone. Mrs. E required help with bathing, meal preparation, medication management, and housekeeping. She could no longer do flower arranging or decorating without assistance, and because getting out was so difficult, she became increasingly housebound.

Without the mental stimulation of being with others, Mrs. E became increasingly paranoid, more and more fearful about new residents in the neighborhood and even the service providers who came to set up her medication trays or deliver meals. Her activities consisted of watching television, cooking an occasional meal, reading the newspaper, poring over catalogs, and talking with her sisters on the phone. She became increasingly isolated.

At 79, Mrs. E had another stroke, which was at least in part brought on by her inability to follow her medication regimen. She was worried about the expense of her medications and would save pills instead of taking them. Her doctors did not expect her to survive this stroke, but she did. During her lengthy recovery, she lived in a nursing home near her daughter, who lived in an adjacent state. Gradually, she recovered her ability to speak and walk with a walker. Because she was in a rich social environment in the nursing home, she also recovered her excellent social skills and made many new friends. The art therapy staff person at the nursing home was encouraging, and Mrs. E discovered an interest in watercolors. Some of her watercolors were featured in local exhibitions. The activities program at the nursing home offered her many opportunities to listen to musical performances, attend religious services, do her art, and keep up with current events—all things she had stopped doing when she was housebound.

Mrs. E and I had the following conversation about a year after her move to the nursing home.

"Do you miss [your former home and community]?" I asked.
"Not really," she replied.
"Would you want to go back?"

"No."

"Why not?"

"I like it here," she said.

"What's so special about here?"

"The people. I have lots of people to help me, I get to do a lot of things I enjoy, I get to see [her daughter and son-in-law] more, and I can still talk to my sisters on the phone. I've made new friends. Art excites me."

At 80, Mrs. E seemed more contented with life than she did at 75. Her case illustrates how a supportive environment can help a person reconstitute continuity. Mrs. E's awakened interest in art, which she sees as related to her earlier activity of flower arranging, is a new spiritual connection for her.

CONCLUSION

In working with elders, we must remember that most elders have two some-what contradictory goals: remaining independent and maintaining their social network. Often, to maintain the social network means having to accept help both in getting out and in bringing people in. The need to be independent and self-reliant, which is so important to most people, can become a hindrance to good adaptation when disability occurs. Without help, everyday tasks of self-care become so energy- and time-intensive that they are all-consuming and leave little in the way of resources for activities that maintain quality of life. One way to work with this situation is to include social elements in care plans. Being in the flow of art or music is not of instrumental value in terms of meeting the body's needs, but it can nourish the soul. And both art and music can have the advantage of not being dependent on verbal ability. Thus, they are not just activities designed to keep people busy. They can also have spiritual and healing qualities.

Continuity theory can help us map the personal systems of those we serve. By asking careful questions about what has been important to persons in the past, we can see how to help them see ways to realize their underlying values in the present. However, we cannot expect them to voluntarily turn their back on a life structure that has served them well in the past. That is why most people cannot see anything good about moving to an assisted living or nursing home setting. They need help in seeing continuity in their life before and after the move. Most fundamentally, continuity resides in the values that inform choice, not just in the specifics of everyday environments and activities.

I have painted an optimistic picture of aging and the human spirit based on my thirty-five years of research on adaptation to various aspects of aging. I have gained tremendous respect for the people I have studied, for their magnificent insights and capabilities. I also have great admiration for their capacity to prevail in the face of what sometimes seem insurmountable difficulties. My main points are that continuity of values, attitudes, lifestyles, and relationships, as well as spiritual development in later adulthood, provide most people with robust resources for coping with changing circumstances and also provide a sense of direction.

To be of help to elders, we can benefit from having a framework within which we can learn about their personal systems. Those who work with elders can use these perspectives to discover and support their clients' aspirations for the last stages of life.

Continuity and spiritual growth are robust resources that see most people through the aging process. But disability and a thinning social network can create a need to reconfigure the personal system. Many people need outreach services that accompany and support them as they modify their personal system to their new circumstances. Continuity and spiritual development are helpful in this process, too.

CHAPTER SEVEN

Spiritual Beliefs and Practices and the Experience of Time and Aging

> Time has two aspects. There is the arrow, the running
> river, without which there is no change, no progress, or
> direction, or creation. And there is the circle or cycle,
> without which there is chaos, meaningless succession of
> instants, a world without clocks or seasons or promises.
> —*Ursula K. LeGuin*

> Time is not a road—it is a room.   —*John Fowles*

This chapter is about the influence of spiritual beliefs and practices on the experience of time as people age. To deal effectively with this complex topic, we must look briefly at several meanings of time and at why the experience of chronological time might accelerate with age. Then we can examine spiritual beliefs about time and practices that might affect perceptions of time. Finally, we can consider how spiritual beliefs and practices might mediate the relationship between age and the experience of time.

Life is too short. This common saying is seldom uttered by young people; it is used by middle-aged and older people to indicate that time is precious and that we cannot afford to waste it, especially on interpersonal conflicts or frustrating activities. But the experience of time depends on the context, which includes age and spiritual beliefs and practices.

Experiential time can be fast or slow; it is relative. As Albert Einstein said, "When you sit with a nice girl for two hours, you think it's only a minute. But when you sit on a hot stove for a minute, you think it's two hours. That's relativity" (Safransky 1990, 49). The subjective nature of experienced time does not mean that it is not affected by social and cultural influences. Indeed, like most personal mental constructs, the meaning of time is conditioned by social norms and expectations.

Historical time stretches back at least five thousand years in the written record and forward as far as the mind can project, but this sense of the word *year* is different from the meaning we attach to a calendar year because we can experience the passing of a calendar year whereas we cannot experience a millennium. Unless we transcend our own potential lifetime in our view of the future, we cannot think about the needs of future generations. Being able to think in panoramic time is thus an important human skill.

We are all tied to the various biological clocks within our bodies that influence the processes of senescence. We experience the effects of these biological clocks, such as gradual stiffening of joints in later adulthood, even though they operate outside our consciousness and therefore outside our experience.

By contrast, we are constantly made aware of chronological time because it is used to order our lives. Unlike preliterate societies, which tended to use rough measures of time, based mostly on movement of the sun, phases of the moon, change of seasons, and annual cycles of animal and plant life, modern and postmodern societies are fixated on chronological time. Most of us carry devices strapped to our wrists that allow us to know the chronological time reasonably precisely. We use technology to keep our room temperature constant across the seasons and to light our environments at all hours of the day and night, which allows us to ignore the natural rhythms of daylight and darkness. Our lives are organized around a time to arise, a time to go to work, time schedules at work, times to eat, times for prayer, times for recreation, and a time for sleep. Constructing an ideal lifestyle in today's world could be expected to include a daily routine tied to the clock. Clock time is used so extensively to organize our many activities that few people can get by without a time-planning device such as a detailed calendar.

In addition to hourly, daily, seasonal, and annual cycles of time, the cultural life course sets forth general chronological age ranges at which we are expected to move from one life stage to another. Thus, most people enter middle age around age 40, later adulthood around age 60, and old age around 80. These cultural life stages are composite pictures of lifestyles and values that are expected of persons in a particular life stage. Most people go through the various life-stage transitions on schedule, chronologically.

Despite the heavy emphasis on chronological time in our culture, most people are aware that our perceptions of the speed of time's passing are not mechanistic but depend on what we are experiencing during a given span of chronological time. The conventional wisdom has it that, with advancing age, time is experienced as accelerating, to the point that by age 90 the years seem to go by rapidly. Most aging individuals report that this generally fits their experience. Possible explanations for this phenomenon are several. First, individuals may be so overhabituated that nothing novel seems to happen in their lives,[1] which in turn may give them few experiential referents from which to estimate the speed of time's passage. Second, as people are freed from child-rearing and regular employment, they may be liberated from the tyranny of the clock. As a result, they may no longer be intensely sensitive to the passage of time; they may not pay as much attention to time. Third, it is possible that the activities that engage elders are more susceptible to what Mihaly Csziks-szentmihalyi (1990) calls "flow," one characteristic of which is losing track of the passage of time. Fourth, as people grow older, accomplishing routine tasks may take longer, and what once was a comfortable daily routine may now seem time pressured. These all seem reasonable explanations for why time is perceived to pass more quickly as age increases.

However, there is also evidence that both belief and behavior can influence perceptions. What we *believe* to be true, we are more apt to *perceive* to be true, and vice versa. For example, if we believe that sane people can experience visions, then we may be more likely to interpret an experience of an angel as a vision rather than a hallucination. Likewise, if we continue to practice in an area of life, our perceptions can be influenced by what we learn from our practice. For example, musicians must learn a complex process of creating rhythm and timing in music. As they continue to practice, their experiences of both producing rhythm and listening to rhythm can change over time. Young musicians often seem to be trying to create the largest possible number of notes for a given time period, whereas older musicians often pay more attention to the beauty available by alternating periods of sound and silence into a simpler, more elegant rhythm.

Studies of how aging might influence the experience of time have thus far ignored the spiritual aspects of being human. However, it is likely that both spiritual beliefs about time and spiritual practices over time influence the relation between aging and the experience of time.

As in earlier chapters, I use *spiritual* here to refer to beliefs, practices, and experiences that loosely revolve around an inner domain of human experience. Spiritual experience includes sensory and psychological input but extends to include transcendent ways of knowing as well.

To develop understanding of how aging interacts with the experience of time and how this relationship may be mediated by spiritual beliefs and practices requires concepts about the many relationships among aging, spirituality, and time. We will illustrate how this might be done by selectively reviewing beliefs about the meaning of time in various spiritual traditions, by discussing the relationship between various spiritual practices and the experience of time, and by looking at how spiritual beliefs and practices might mediate the relationship between aging and the experience of time.

BELIEFS ABOUT TIME

Important beliefs about time include whether or not there is a continuation of personal consciousness after death, whether elders are obligated to take a panoramic view of time in order to lead the society into the future, whether life stages are related to inner spiritual growth, and whether inner spiritual growth changes the experience of time. Does spiritual growth include a timeless state of consciousness in which the experience of time does not exist? Does spiritual growth require focus on transcendent experience, present-moment awareness, or both? How does the focus of awareness affect experiences of time?

Belief in a personal afterlife is characteristic of many religious belief systems, and belief in a personal afterlife means that the life span of one's human body is but a tiny fraction of the time available, which downplays the importance of the current lifetime. Likewise, belief in an afterlife in another life form through reincarnation minimizes the importance of getting it right within one lifetime. By contrast, some religions contend that this is it, you only go around once, and time in the current lifetime is therefore more important than for those who believe in eternal life in some particular form. If people believe in one lifetime, then approaching the end of that lifetime can produce much more powerful spiritual growth as well as despair at lack of growth. For example, perceiving that there is not enough time left to perfect the self can be an important motive for letting go of perfectionism and being able to integrate the ideal self with the real self, with its range of good and bad qualities and history. Of course, even people who believe in an afterlife may face an existential crisis when physical death becomes real to them if they have not converted their belief into the certainty of faith.

Young and middle-aged adults are often expected to focus their attention on relatively short-range goals, such as getting a formal education, maintaining a connection with the economy, selecting a life partner and rearing children, and contributing their energies to the community. Leaders of business, government, and voluntary organizations develop five-year plans, not hundred-year plans. But Zalman Schachter-Shalomi and Ronald Miller (1995) make the point that elders are uniquely qualified to take the long view. Child launching and retirement, a long span of experienced historical time, with its many changes, and feelings of generativity about the welfare of grandchildren and great-grandchildren are interests that motivate elders to be concerned about what sort of world we will be leaving for our offspring over the next hundred years. To Schachter-Shalomi and Miller, this perspective leads to greater concern over the welfare of the planet Earth, especially its environmental, intercultural, and political integrity. Elders traditionally played this role, but in the process of modernization this role was transferred to "experts," who often do not look at issues from a panoramic time perspective. *Spiritual Eldering* is the expression Zalman Schachter-Shalomi and Ronald Miller use to indicate that recovering the role of elder in postmodern societies requires a level of spiritual development on the part of elders before they can have the transcendent attitudes and panoramic view of time required to play the role of spiritual elder.

Many faith traditions relate spiritual development to stages of the life course. For example, the Hindu conception of life stages includes a householder stage and a renunciate stage. In the householder stage, people use their concern with family and vocation to motivate an inner spiritual journey involving meditation, not as an escape from reality but as a way of seeing ultimate truth in their everyday lives. In the renunciate stage, which traditionally began with the birth of the first grandson, people do not drop out of life to become recluses. Instead, they become so focused on the Absolute within themselves that they gain a transcendent perspective that allows them to see themselves and their world in a different way, a way in which time is fully understood as a human creation. From an experiential point of view, time is in you, you are not in time.

This basic Hindu philosophical position was used by Lars Tornstam to develop his theory of gerotranscendence (Tornstam 2005). He posited that advanced aging increases interest in contemplation, which in turn produces a shift in perspective that dramatically reduces the importance of chronological time. Thus, one might argue that the loosening of social constraints that occurs in later adulthood and old age allows contemplative understanding to blossom into transcendence, with a dramatic effect on the experience of time. Note that these are *concepts* of the relation between aging, life stage, spirituality, and the experience of time.

Thomas Cole (1992) provided an insightful portrait of how biblical ideas from Jewish and Christian perspectives shaped early American Protestant conceptions of the relation between life stages and spiritual development. Old age was seen as the culmination of a spiritual journey of life. Elders, through their lifelong struggle to understand and carry out the will of God, were more developed spiritually compared with the young. That is, experience across time was assumed to be a necessary element of spiritual insight. Elders were expected to set a moral and social example for the young. Early American religion had high expectations of elders, including dignified behavior and appearance and continued social contribution. These ideas are very much a part of the life course expectations in American churches today.

But these ideas of spiritual growth over time compete with a view that the effects of aging—whether aging means growing decrepitude and incapacity or continued vitality—are largely under the individual's moral control. And the evangelical view of salvation as immediately wiping away sin means that the experience of elders is downplayed. The notion of respect for elders remains, but a sense that elders, by virtue of their experience of contemplation and struggle, can be spiritually advanced, is often missing.

Concepts of time, and therefore of aging, as being needed for spiritual growth can be a sometime thing, depending on the directions of cultural change. By the year 2000, religious thought was again becoming more open to the image of spiritual growth with aging. This trend is no doubt related to more cultural emphasis having been placed on the positive aspects of aging during the 1990s. It is also probably related to the greater attention in popular culture and gerontology research to the voices of experience, to the journals and oral histories produced by elders themselves, which often contain commentaries about how extended life experience relates to spiritual insight.

Most religious traditions also contain beliefs about the effects of transcendence and present-moment awareness on the experience of time. For example, although the major concepts of Jewish, Christian, and Islamic traditions are all rooted in a personified conception of God, there are within each of these traditions mystical, experiential concepts of God, not as person-like but as mysterious and capable of being only incompletely apprehended by the verbal mind. For instance, in *The Cloud of Unknowing* (Anon. 2004), perhaps the first Christian meditation guide to have been originally written in the English language, the anonymous fourteenth-century author holds that God is obscured by a "cloud of unknowing," which can be navigated only by assuming an open stance of bare being. The cloud of unknowing is within the experiencer, not something external, but to even sense the cloud of unknowing, the meditator must leave worldly concerns, including time, behind in a "cloud of forgetting." This conception of God is similar to the Hindu conception of the Absolute. Eternal God, or Absolute, is not characterized by infinite time but by an absence of time. Thus, if people connect with the experience of God or the Absolute within themselves, they transcend time as well as the other aspects of a phenomenal world bound by concepts such as time and space. As Ken Wilber (2001, 148) put it, "The Absolute can be present in its entirety at every point in time only if [the Absolute] is itself timeless." This same general perspective is contained in the Buddhist concept of nothingness, which is less an absence or void than no-thing-ness; not this, not that, but an entirety in which ideas such as subject/object, time, and space do not apply.

To experience "the ground of being," Aldous Huxley's (1944) term for the ultimate principle that forms the eternal context for spiritual experience, thus requires that we transcend conventional consciousness. A major obstacle to transcendence is being distracted by worldly concerns. Although it may be possible by strength of will to develop the skill needed to be "in the world but not of it" early in life, transcendence is thought to be more common in later life, for the reasons mentioned above.

Paradoxically, aging is also thought to make possible a greater capacity to be in the present. Although stereotypes hold that elders dwell excessively in the past, my research has shown that healthy elders living in the community experience a balance of thoughts and experiences from the past, present, and future (Atchley 1999). Indeed, the proportion of elders who have the capacity to patiently attend to the present with present-moment awareness is much greater than that of young and middle-aged adults. Present-moment awareness is also a form of timelessness, in the sense that the present moment, not the passage of time, is of the essence.

SPIRITUAL PRACTICES AND THE EXPERIENCE OF TIME

Various religious traditions contain rituals that are designed to break the hold of the everyday world on consciousness. For instance, the Jewish concept of the Sabbath is more than just a day of rest; it is a time for renewing one's

relationship with God. The Muslim practice of daily prayer creates five opportunities each day—on arising, at midday, in mid-afternoon, at sunset, and
when retiring for the evening—to focus attention on the divine. Catholic mo-
nastic traditions schedule breaks for prayer and contemplation seven times
each day: at daybreak, around 9 am, at noon, at 3 pm, about 6 pm, in the
early evening, and at midnight. Most meditation-based traditions encourage
practitioners to have a specific time for meditation each day in order to make
meditation a habit. These rituals all use concepts of time to create pauses in
the swirl of worldly activities, pauses during which attention can be focused
on ultimate concerns.

The discipline of regular spiritual practice over time creates a rhythm of
connection with the ground of being, and this rhythm can become a self-sus-
taining system in the sense that, in all their variety, the experiences that come
from spiritual practice become ends in themselves. Over time, contemplative
prayer and meditation may become less means to an end and more ends in
themselves, and in most cases this occurs over an extended period of time.

Meditation is a central spiritual practice in many spiritual traditions. Unfortunately, the word *meditation* often evokes a stereotype of people dressed
in flowing robes and sitting in the lotus position. People confuse the outer appearance for the inner intention. In fact, there are many different meditation
methods, and individuals may use one or several of them, depending on their
immediate needs. How various meditation practices influence the experience
of time varies greatly. For example, the Transcendental Meditation technique
uses meditation on a mantra—subvocal sounds that have been found to focus
attention—to induce a transcendent state of consciousness that is completely
beyond sensory and verbal experience. In this state, the meditator loses track
of time completely. On the other hand, Buddhist mindfulness meditation involves paying close attention to sensations of breathing, which focuses attention on simply being rather than on what the body or the mind may be
doing. In the beginning, mindfulness meditators often experience the passage
of time as excruciatingly slow. But after years of daily meditation and intensive meditation retreats, practitioners tend to "give up on time." As conscious
being becomes a larger and larger part of the mindfulness meditation experience, which takes time, time often matters less during meditation.

Prayer is also a central spiritual practice for most faith traditions. Prayer
can be classified into ritual prayer, petitionary prayer, and meditative prayer.
Ritual prayer, repeated over and over for countless repetitions, can have transcendental effects, carrying the practitioner out of conventional conscious-

ness and into greater sensitivity to the divine. But ritual prayer can also induce a devotional attitude toward God or serve as a reminder of important religious or spiritual ideas. Petitionary prayer asks something of God. Meditative prayer has little form. The practitioner simply "waits upon the Lord." The point is to be present, open, attuned to messages from God, yet not expecting any specific experience. James Peacock and Margaret Paloma (1991) found that younger adults were much more likely to engage in ritual and petitionary prayer compared with older adults, and older adults were much more likely to engage in meditative prayer compared with younger adults. In my twenty-year longitudinal study of adults who were age 70 and older at the completion of the study, I found that the incidence of contemplative prayer increased substantially with age.

Meditation and prayer are spiritual practices that tend to work mostly with the mind and basic consciousness. However, movement disciplines such as tai chi or dance, music, and other arts can also be important spiritual practices. As spiritual practices, expressive disciplines can invoke what Cszikszentmihalyi (1990) calls "flow," which is experienced as an intense and effortless concentration wherein there is no experience of time. Thus, as spiritual practices, these activities can require intense attention to the present moment; they can also transcend time.

SPIRITUAL BELIEFS AND PRACTICES, AGING, AND THE EXPERIENCE OF TIME

Virtually none of the studies of changes in how the passage of time is perceived as one ages has been able to look at individual differences that might be attributable to spiritual beliefs and practices because these studies did not assess individual spiritual beliefs and practices. In this section, I look at some possibilities that might be useful for future inquiry.

How might spiritual beliefs and practices mediate the relation between aging and the experience of time? First, such mediation might occur as a result of the effects of spiritual beliefs and practices on the potential causes of altered time perception with age.

For example, some perceptions of a speed-up in time with age may be a result of paying less attention to time through overhabituation or the experience of flow. If overhabituation is a cause of the perception that time accelerates with age, then mindfulness practice could be expected to offset this tendency. The practice of mindfulness meditation involves intense awareness of the details of the present moment. Mindfulness is the opposite of overhabituation, and in mindfulness people perceive their environment more intensely than in conventional consciousness. In a state of mindfulness, people are intensely focused on the present moment and not preoccupied with time.

Even people who are overhabituated may find that spiritual practice takes them to a region of consciousness in which time is irrelevant and therefore not perceived as passing quickly. For example, people who engage in ritual prayer for long periods each day or who spend much of their time in contemplation might be unlikely to perceive the pace of time as important. This would be especially likely in those whose practices emphasize being rather than doing. On the other hand, spiritual practices that emphasize repeated ritual might increase the potential for a "good" type of overhabituation. For example, people who spend hours each day in ritual prayer may be in a pleasant state during this time but still be left with the question, "Where did the time go?"

To the extent that spiritual practices promote an experience of losing oneself in the activity, a process called flow, they take the practitioner to a world unbounded by time. Not all practices that produce the sense of flow are spiritual, but most spiritual practices have the potential for flow. Of course, to be able to ignore time, people must be free to some extent from social time constraints.

If perceiving time as passing quickly is a function of paying less attention to it, then later life offers many opportunities to free life's schedules from "the tyranny of the clock." Retired people often report that they experience a much more relaxed pace and more freedom from time pressures compared with when they were working. People who have launched their children into adulthood often experience a dramatic increase in "free time."

Where the spiritual journey may be involved here is in influencing what people do with the time freed by retirement and the empty nest. Those who use this time for contemplative reading, meditation, prayer, or devotions are choosing a lifestyle that emphasizes an inner journey in a region of consciousness in which time is less relevant. For example, a man in his 80s reported to me, "You become free of time when you realize that time is in you, not you in time."

On the other hand, those who use the time freed by retirement and child launching to become more involved in a path of service may find that they have substituted one set of time-based obligations for another. But time pressures are subjective, and those who have been on a contemplative spiritual path for many years may be able to engage in service without feeling the pressures of time because they take a mindful approach to service, which promotes realistic expectations of what can be accomplished and a let-be attitude toward time.

If aging causes people to slow down, even though they want to continue in their customary lifestyle, then aging may cause an increase in time pressure and a sense that time is speeding up. Many older people drastically simplify their lifestyles in order to balance their capabilities with their expectations. The spiritual journey can have an effect here by altering a person's sense of priorities. As people grow spiritually, they tend to take a transpersonal view of life. They often deemphasize their social and materialistic goals in favor of more enduring inner qualities, such as altruism and generativity.

Beliefs can also mediate the relationship between time and aging. If people believe that their fundamental being is timeless, then death is less fearsome and there is little reason to feel that time is running out, which could be expected to reduce the sense that time is speeding up. On the other hand, if people believe that death is final and that time is finite, as they get older they may begin to see time as a scarce resource and to see it as passing faster.

If people believe in a personal afterlife, time is irrelevant in that their life is eternal. However, if they believe that eternity will be spent either in heaven or hell and that what they do in this life determines which, they may have a heightened sense that time is running out and that time is passing ever more quickly.

If people believe that transcendence and enlightenment are possible, they may experience these states. People who have transcended their purely personal concerns are unlikely to be concerned about the pace at which time passes, regardless of their chronological age.

These various possibilities by no means exhaust the potential ways that spiritual beliefs and practices might mediate the relationship between aging and the perception of time. They do illustrate a complex web of possibilities. As we continue to ask the types of question raised in this book, we will continue to find that spiritual beliefs and practices have important influences.

I have found it useful to think about human beings as interactive systems in which bodily systems, knowledge, mental capacities, coping styles, lifestyles, and social environments interact in complex ways and evolve by incorporating feedback from experience. From this point of view, physical, psychological, and social characteristics are basic structures and processes. Beliefs and practices of individuals are imbedded in a culture and a society, and change in the individual or in the culture or society can change beliefs or practices. But changing beliefs or practices can also affect physical, psychological, or social characteristics, and widespread individual changes in belief or practice can change culture and social arrangements.

Given that a multitude of specific elements is subsumed under the labels of beliefs, practices, aging, and adult development, the number of potential interactions is astronomical. Even if we confine ourselves to the experience of time as affected by physical, psychological, and social aging and adult development, especially spiritual development, the number of potential dimensions to explore is mind-boggling.

CONCLUSION

This chapter begins with a particular general finding in gerontology: aging is often accompanied by a perception that time goes by faster and faster, especially in later life. The relationship between aging and the experience of time might well be conditioned by spiritual beliefs and practices in several important ways. Thus, the chapter illustrates how concepts about spirituality might help us understand variations from this generalization about aging and the experience of time. The logic of this analysis could be used to examine the mediating effects of spirituality on a wide variety of other general findings in gerontology.

CHAPTER EIGHT

Spirituality and the Experience of Dying and Death

What difference does spirituality make in the experience of dying and death? How do dying and death influence spirituality? Those are the central questions for this chapter. Of course, the answers to these questions are deeply influenced by how we answer two other questions: What is my spiritual nature? Am I a person having spiritual experiences or am I a spiritual being having a human experience?

No topic in this chapter has been adequately studied. The ideas here are suggestions about issues that might be studied and how one might think about them and communicate about them. Intellectually, we know that everyone dies, but as Ernest Becker (1973) pointed out long ago, people tend not to like this idea, and many societies and cultures have gone to great lengths to deny that death is real. Many cultural beliefs deny the reality of death by describing in detail a world to which we pass when our time on this earthly plane has ended. Becker felt that these many versions of an afterlife served a single function—to relieve the inevitable anxiety associated with death of the personal self.

What we believe about both the existence and nature of an afterlife and conditions for a smooth transition can profoundly influence our experience when we think about our own death. People who believe that personality and self somehow transcend their body and continue into an afterlife in some kind of personal form, and that a virtuous life leads to heaven while an unvirtuous life leads to hell, may fear death if they are uncertain about whether, as persons, they are virtuous enough to receive the reward of heaven. By contrast, people who see God as an "infinite sea of being" from which they were spiritually born may see death as a gentle releasing back into that infinite sea, not as a person but as nonembodied life energy.

Spiritual experiences can give us confidence in cultural beliefs about death or take confidence away, depending on the match between these experiences and the substance of our beliefs about death. Consider these examples.[1]

Annie was a long-time meditator who had directly experienced the "Absolute" within herself many times. She saw spaceless and timeless being as familiar and unthreatening territory. She did not fear personal death. She saw death as "going home." By age 88, Annie was blind, nearly deaf, and severely crippled by painful arthritis. She had fallen several times and was unable to transfer from her wheelchair without assistance. By her account, her life had become one of sameness and pain. Annie summoned her many friends and told them that she was ready to die. She asked them to accompany her on this last journey. After a ceremonial celebration of Annie's life, Annie ceased taking liquids. Her goal was to die as painlessly as possible. Her friends took shifts being with her around the clock. The first day without fluid was the hardest for Annie, but after that she was peaceful and lucid throughout. After five days, Annie was weak but radiant just before she lost consciousness, and several of her friends were with her two days later when she took her last breath.

⊕

Koji was a 60-year-old Japanese man whose family was Buddhist, but he was not a practicing Buddhist. When he was diagnosed with pancreatic cancer and given only a short time to live, Koji was overcome by a consuming terror. He believed that he would be entering "the Void," but he had no experience of this place. To him it seemed a great unknown. When he thought about his impending death, he experienced a numbing anxiety throughout his body. His wife would sit with him for long periods as this usually taciturn man repeated "I don't want to die—I don't want to die" over and over again like a mantra. Nothing seemed to comfort him. He remained terrified to the end. His lack of spiritual experience or religious faith gave him no possibility of resources from these areas to help him cope.

⊕

Kenneth believed that Christ was his personal savior and that as long as Kenneth held this belief, his sins would be forgiven and he would be assured a personal afterlife in heaven. When he was young, Kenneth had believed this cognitively, but by his 60s he felt it "in his bones." For him, this was not a cliché, it was real. At 71, Kenneth was diagnosed with ALS, commonly called Lou Gehrig's disease, which is a progressive deterioration of nerve functioning throughout the body. ALS often involves a long and painful progression before it finally shuts the body down. Kenneth's belief that he was assured of going to heaven was a great comfort to him through four years of suffering. He said, "I try to remember that the pain and inability to do things is temporary and to see Jesus looking at me with incredible love and I know that soon I will be with Him." Kenneth's positive and hopeful perspective inspired those who took care of him.

Sarah grew up Methodist. She attended church regularly throughout her life, and her faith grew and deepened over time. Familiar hymns and sermons on familiar biblical topics and a community of like-minded people gave Sarah a deep sense of well-being. She made sure that her daughter Julia, an only child, regularly attended Sunday school, and Sarah said prayers with Julia at bedtime each night. When she was 10, Julia was abducted and murdered. Sarah was devastated. She could not reconcile this happening with any conception she had of God. The culprit was never found, and Sarah focused her anger and desolation on God. She took this event as proof that God does not exist; heaven does not exist; only bleakness exists. Three years after Julia's death, Sarah's husband left. Sarah tried many forms of counseling and took antidepressants, but she never regained a sense of well-being. Forty-three years later, when Sarah died, she found no comfort in either spirituality or religion. She saw death as a release from the "flatness" that had been her life since Julia died. She met death with relief, but not hope.

Why some people seek refuge in spirituality and religion during difficult times and others reject spirituality and religion in response to extreme happenings is a mystery.

DYING AND DEATH AS SPIRITUAL JOURNEYS

Cultural concepts of the "good death" vacillate back and forth between acceptance of death and a battle against death. Thomas Cole (1992) describes nineteenth-century concepts of "edifying" death as a process of enlightenment that occurs if one does one's death properly. Most scholars consider this a comforting romanticization of death,[2] but recently a movement has emerged to encourage "conscious dying."

Conscious dying is rooted in the "consciousness movement" that began in the 1940s and gained prominence in popular culture in the late 1960s. Higher states of consciousness and awareness were presumed to be unrealized human potentials. Eastern philosophy and spiritual practices were seen as being especially useful in cultivating inner mystical experiences of higher states. But by the 1970s, early Christian sources, such as *The Cloud of Unknowing* and the writings of St. John of the Cross and St. Teresa of Avila, were supporting Christians on mystical inner journeys.

In 1982, Stephen Levine published *Who Dies? An Investigation of Conscious Living and Conscious Dying*, which quickly became a central resource for people who wanted to integrate what they had been learning from the consciousness movement with issues of dying and death. It also introduced many people who worked with dying people to the consciousness movement.

One of the central themes of Eastern philosophy is that to progress spiritually we must come to terms with aging and death. As long as we deny or repress aging and death, we cannot experience our true nature as spiritual beings. Conscious dying starts with the premise that to be fully conscious as we die we must learn to center our awareness in consciousness—in pure being, not in our minds and not in our bodies. Awareness centered in the mind leads to fear of decline and extinction of the mind. To move awareness away from exclusive focus on the mind, loosening our attachment to the mind can be helpful. Awareness centered in the body can lead to preoccupation with decline and loss of physical capacities. To move awareness away from exclusive focus on the body, relaxing our clinging attachment to the body can help. If we see our existence as being made up of being, embodiment, and consciousness, then concerns about the health of body and mind can be seen as appropriate because they serve the whole. But preoccupation with physical existence or thought can be seen as unhealthy because it is not balanced by beingness.

The concept of conscious dying presumes that dying experienced from higher states of consciousness is less likely to lead to fear or anxiety compared with dying experienced from excessive concerns with preserving one's body or personality. Aging can often be an ally in adopting a detached attitude about the body and mind. As people age, they often learn to be philosophically accepting of losses they can do nothing about, and this detachment from body and mind can encourage spiritual development in later life. The research on gerotranscendence (Atchley 1999; Tornstam 2005) indicates that, for most people, aging is accompanied by reduced fear of death.

As we saw in Chapter 6, continuity and spiritual development are important resources for coping with challenges of later life, and this is particularly true of dying. Continuity of spirituality, values, and relationships is especially helpful as support, and spiritual development leads toward a higher place from which to view one's dying.

WHAT HAPPENS AT THE MOMENT OF DEATH?

No one knows for sure what happens when we die, but most of us have come to at least a working conclusion about this event. The evidence we have comes mainly from reports given by people who have had near-death experiences, who have been thought dead or pronounced dead but who have been revived. Consistencies across near-death reports include feelings of peace, feelings of painlessness, hearing strange sounds, out-of-body experience, seeing light or beings of light, and reluctance to return to the body (Raymond Moody 1975; Williams 2005). This list brings to mind the following quote from Huxley: "Lightly, my darling, lightly, even when it comes to dying. Nothing ponderous or portentous or emphatic. No rhetoric, no tremolos, no self-conscious persona putting on its celebrated imitation of Christ, or Goethe, or Little Nell. And of course, no theology, no metaphysics. Just the simple fact of dying and the fact of the clear light" (quoted in Levine 1982, 249). However, a small proportion (12%) of respondents in a 1982 Gallup Poll reported that their near-death experience involved torment, not peace (www.gallup.com).

Many people who have near-death experiences say that the experience changed them, usually from people preoccupied with matters of achievement and material gain to people concerned with helping others. One could take this as evidence that near-death experiences take people to a higher state of consciousness, which puts conventional values into a different perspective.

DEATH AS SPIRITUAL TRANSITION AND BELIEF IN AN AFTERLIFE

The Tibetan Buddhists exemplify a highly organized approach to preparing for a death that is seen as a complex passage. They believe that following physical death we enter an intermediate state of being as we await rebirth. In this intermediate state, we begin by having spiritual clarity associated with death and then we experience terrifying hallucinations arising from the impulses of one's previous unmindful actions, often called karma. Tibetan Buddhists believe that a dead person can be helped in this transition by hearing inspirational words that draw awareness toward clarity rather than toward karmic impulses. Thus, for several days after death, friends and family sit with the dead body and read helpful texts. Tibetan Buddhists prepare for death by becoming familiar with these texts so that they will recognize them when they hear them after death.

Roman Catholic Christians believe that persons who die with only pardonable sins that have not been absolved do not go to hell but go instead to purgatory, where they are purged of their sins until they reach the absolute purity required to enter heaven. People who follow this doctrine could be expected to be motivated to have as few unrepented sins as possible so as to minimize their time in the "fires" of purgatory.

Obviously, whether we see death as a spiritual transition or not depends on beliefs about the existence and nature of an afterlife and the conditions required for a smooth passage from this life to the next. (See Kastenbaum [2004] for a comprehensive discussion of the enormous variety of beliefs concerning death and afterlife.) Research on fear of death suggests that from the viewpoint of a dying person, the specifics of these beliefs are not as important as the person's *confidence* in them. Atheists who were confident that death means just ceasing to exist were likely to be unafraid of death. Religious people who were confident in their beliefs about an afterlife were equally likely to be unafraid of death. However, people who were unsure in their beliefs about death were the most likely to experience a high degree of fear and anxiety about death (Koenig 1995).

My hypothesis is that for many people spiritual experiences are a resource in deciding the plausibility of various scenarios about the nature of death and an afterlife. For example, if a person has experienced higher levels of consciousness as being nonpersonal, it may be difficult to accept beliefs about an afterlife in which one remains a person and interacts with persons in one's family or with friends who have died. On the other hand, if a person has experienced having conversations with the personal spirits of friends or family members who have died, then beliefs in personal continuity into an afterlife may be more plausible.

EXISTENTIAL INFLUENCES ON THE EXPERIENCE OF DYING AND DEATH

The extent to which death is seen as an unknown is related to opportunities to see people die and to see the dead. These opportunities are not randomly distributed in the population and depend partly on regional, ethnic, and cultural influences, including social class. For example, where people die, whether the body is displayed, how (naturally, or embalmed and cosmetically presented) and where (home, funeral home, or church), and the existence and content of memorial services all have the potential to influence attitudes toward death and to stimulate spiritual experiences associated with death.

In American society, death is mostly experienced in the media. On television and in movies we may see dozens of people who are fictionally "dead" for every actually dead person, and even pictures of the truly dead do not have the immediacy of seeing someone die and be dead. Consider an experience I had as a child.

By the time I was ten, I had seen many people "die" in the movies, and these same people were miraculously "resurrected" for the next grade B shoot-'em-up. One Saturday I was walking home from the movies and saw a woman hit by a car. Her body was catapulted high in the air, hit a tree limb, and she landed on her head on the sidewalk about thirty feet in front of me. Her skull was caved in and a large pool of blood formed. Her eyes were half open and vacant. I stood stunned on the sidewalk for only a minute or so before someone came out of a nearby barber shop and placed an apron over the woman's upper body. One minute she was walking across the street and the next instant she was dead.

This experience drove home the reality of physical death for me. Seeing this real and sudden death forced me to think about what happens when people die in a way that none of the fictional deaths I had seen in the movies had. At that time in my life, although I attended a Baptist church, I was attending a parochial Catholic school, and we were studying about purgatory in religion class. I wondered if this woman would go to hell or if she would go to purgatory. I doubted that she would go straight to heaven, because I had learned in school that even saints are not pure enough to go to heaven without first being purged of sin. I asked my mother about this that evening, and she said, "I imagine she's in a better place now." I took this to mean that Mom thought the woman was in heaven. So this experience not only altered my view of the fact of death, it brought me into direct contact with religious differences in the meaning of death and conditions for experiencing an afterlife. I liked the idea of assuming that people would go to heaven unless you had evidence to the contrary.

By the time people reach later life, they have usually had many experiences that require them to cope with the contradictions and paradoxes about death and an afterlife that exist in our American cultural soup.

CONCERNS ABOUT DYING AND QUALITY OF LIFE

The greatest fear about dying is that we will lose control over the circumstances of our dying and be forced to endure pain, suffering, and indignities we did not choose. Many more people fear this than fear death itself (Atchley and Barusch 2004). One of the greatest benefits of being part of a spiritual community is confidence that if the need arises, there will be people to accompany you on your final journey who share your spiritual perspective on dying and who will intercede on your behalf with health care providers whose agendas may conflict with yours.

However, we should not assume that people are helpless in the face of the medical-industrial complex. Here are two examples in which aging people took charge of the conditions of their dying.

Being a close friend or immediate family member often provides an opportunity to be intensely involved in another person's dying process. In the mid-1990s I was part of the dying process of Millie, my best friend and colleague of more than twenty-five years, and Gar, my wife's beloved father. These two endings were different in duration and circumstances, but I was struck by the ways in which both were able to influence their experience of dying.

At 81, Gar seemed in good general health, but he was a long-time smoker and had mild diabetes. He suffered congestive heart failure in the early evening at home. Gar told the EMTs to let him die. But guidelines didn't allow that. Instead, Gar was transported by helicopter to a large medical complex a half-day's drive away. Gar kept saying, "I don't want to go."

Three days later, the doctors at the medical center convinced the family that with a coronary artery bypass and heart-valve replacement, Gar could probably enjoy several more years of good health. Gar was not so sure, especially after the staff required him to watch a video graphically showing all the things they were asking his permission to do to his body. I noticed that at several points during the video, Gar's attention was obviously elsewhere. But in the end, mostly to please his family—I think, Gar gave his consent.

While the surgical team was beginning anesthesia, Gar suddenly went into cardiac arrest. They performed CPR on him. Some time later, a visibly shaken surgeon came to tell us, "We lost him, and frankly I don't understand what happened."

I thought about what Gar had been saying to everyone for three days—that he was ready for his life to be over. No one stood ready to be his ally in this. But in the end, it seemed to me that his intention was more powerful than the wishes of his family or the arsenal of Western medicine. He wanted to leave, and he left.

❋

At 71, Millie was diagnosed with lung cancer, which was treated with surgery and multiple courses of chemotherapy and radiation. She had a period of monitoring and things were looking good, but a follow-up exam revealed that cancer had spread to her bones and from there would invade her entire body. She was told that her dying would take about six months.

In July, as I sit in Millie's bright, airy living room, I become aware that I feel anxious. For the first time in more than twenty-five years of close friendship, I don't know what to say or do. Millie is dying, but it won't happen soon. I am committed to accompanying and serving her as best I can during this last journey, but nothing I have ever done before has prepared me for this moment.

Over the next week or so, I become clearer about what she expects of me. Because she can no longer easily go out into the world, my daily job is delivering a stack of office mail and helping Millie attend to it, but what she really wants is the latest university gossip.

I am part of an intricate division of labor involving more than a dozen close friends and family members Millie has mobilized to meet her needs during her dying. There can be no mistake about it: Millie is in charge and makes the important decisions. I feel enormous relief to be able just to follow instructions.

By early October, Millie seems frail and is in a lot of pain. She frequently appears to be embarrassed about being in pain, as if she doesn't think it is seemly. But there really is no dignified way to be in agony. We sit in silence for long periods. I am beginning to appreciate this silence—almost like group meditation, except Millie would never admit to meditating. I think the peacefulness is helpful to Millie, but we don't speak about it.

In early November, Millie is excited about traveling from Ohio to Atlanta to attend the Gerontological Society of America meetings, where she is scheduled to receive a prestigious award. I look at her and I cannot see how she will be able to withstand the trip. She is weak and emaciated and in intense pain much of the time. But her eyes are bright as she talks about seeing her many professional friends one last time.

The gerontology meeting is a triumph for Millie. Even in her wheelchair, she is resplendent in stylish new clothes and gaucho-style hat. Several hundred colleagues rise to their feet and give her a standing ovation that lasts several minutes. Millie accepts this accolade with grace and humility.

At a reception later that day, a long line of people waits patiently throughout the two-hour event for a few last words with Millie. As always, she is attentive, gracious, and supportive with each person. One colleague says to me, "At first, I was shocked at Millie's appearance. She has changed a lot and seems frail. But then I looked into her eyes, at the fire, and I said to myself, it's the same Millie." I cannot fathom where she is getting the energy to keep this up. I realize later that it is coming from the people who want so much to be with her.

When Millie returns from Atlanta, I go over for my usual visit, and her immediate family members are all there for Thanksgiving. Millie looks tired but is in good spirits. I suggest that I wait until after the holiday to come by again, because she has a lot of company. She gives me an enigmatic look and says, "Call tomorrow."

I call as instructed, and Millie's daughter tearfully tells me that Millie is slipping in and out of consciousness. She dies two days later, at home surrounded by her loving family.

About two weeks after her funeral, Millie's husband calls to say that he needs to deliver something. Millie had spent time during her dying carefully selecting little gifts from among her personal possessions to give to her friends. My gift is a well-used rectangular silver pillbox with a raised figure of the Buddha embossed in the lid. The more I gaze at the worn image, the more it looks like Millie.

LESSONS

Gar's experience fits the stereotype of an older person's having important decisions taken away by doctors and family, but he nevertheless seemed to take control of his own dying through a deep inner process. The lesson is to respect the will to die as much as the will to live.

The high level of control Millie exercised over her dying process did not occur by accident. She consciously and carefully orchestrated her social circumstances to provide herself with the companionship, support, and power she would need for her last journey. She gently and persistently helped family members and friends accept and support her decisions.

Through her strong will, Millie remained in charge of the decisions about her healthcare, and she used her extensive network of knowledgeable friends to carefully select medical practitioners who could support her desire to be in charge of her experience of dying. As a result, she was able to get the palliative care she needed to ease her pain and spend her last months at home. She refused treatment that would have affected her alertness, and she rejected treatment that would have diminished the quality of her life experience. She resisted pressures from her doctors, family, and friends to grasp at medical straws. She conserved her energy for one last important trip, and died at home surrounded by the loving people who knew her best. She had a plan for how and when her life would end, and she died under the circumstances she had prepared for.

Neither Gar nor Millie had strong religious beliefs or ever talked about spiritual experiences. But Gar was a wheat farmer and cattleman for whom nature's wonders were a part of daily life, and he felt connected to the natural world and the land in a profound, unspoken way. He looked at his own death as a natural thing not to be postponed or avoided. Millie was an observant Jew who did not believe in an afterlife, nor did she give much credence to mysticism, but there was an intense aliveness—a beingness—in Millie that hundreds of people saw, wanted to be around, and respected. I have been told by dozens of Millie's friends that they saw her as a spiritual person, but she herself would probably have rejected that label—as any properly humble sage would.

CONCLUSION

The reality of dying and death are catalysts that propel many people to ponder spiritual questions deeply and perhaps begin a spiritual journey. Likewise, spiritual experiences can profoundly affect how we see the prospect of death and the process of dying. Yet the potential ways in which these issues play out in actual lives have not been studied extensively; here is a vast field of research awaiting discovery.

Conclusion

Summary, Reflections, and Implications

I began my study of aging in 1963 in a graduate seminar taught by Clark Tibbitts, one of the founders of social gerontology. As a text, we used the *Handbook of Social Gerontology* (Tibbitts 1960), a thorough compendium of research findings and ideas about social aspects of aging from a wide variety of academic disciplines. In that handbook, there was an excellent chapter by Paul B. Maves, "Aging, Religion, and the Church," which dealt mainly with Jewish and Christian teachings and attitudes toward aging, care of the aged by religious bodies, and participation of elders in churches. Maves concluded that as people age, religion is increasingly a comfort to the extent that it provides answers to "meaning of life" questions and a feeling of safety and security by imposing religious order on the universe. The words *spirituality* or *spiritual* do not appear anywhere in this chapter or handbook; neither were these words used in the companion volume, *Handbook of Aging and the Individual* (Birren 1959). These books accurately reflected the state of the literature of that era. Thus, as a beginning student of gerontology, I had no opportunity to include the concept of spirituality in my studies.

Fortunately, for my dissertation I did face-to-face interviews with more than a hundred older women on the impact of retirement on the self concepts of female teachers and telephone operators. I observed the results of spiritual development in these women. Most of them were lively people who had a clear understanding of themselves and of what was meaningful to them about their lifestyles, well-honed personal value systems built from life experience, and a quiet, strong connection to the sacred within themselves. Many of them used their spiritual worldview and spiritual presence as the basic organizing force in their lifestyles, family lives, and service work in the community. Unfortunately, it took me about fifteen years to gain the vocabulary needed to fully describe what I was observing in these women because gerontology, like most of America, was not paying attention at that time to spirituality as an inner experience or connection to the sacred or to its potential motivating power.

Earlier, I discussed Robert Wuthnow's (1998) argument that since the 1950s spirituality in America shifted from a religion-centered "spirituality of dwelling" toward a person-centered "spirituality of seeking" and later toward a "spirituality of practice." A spirituality of dwelling emphasizes unchanging ritual and organizational structure. Comfort, security, and answers come from predictability. By contrast, a spirituality of seeking emphasizes journeying and negotiation. On a journey we never know exactly what we will confront, but we must remain aware of our needs and pay attention to opportunities in order to meet our changing circumstances. On the spiritual journey, we never have perfect maps, so we need an enduring set of questions that will allow us to discover the ground of being in that time and place.

Wuthnow (1998) argues that most people live a life that balances dwelling and seeking; they like the security of dwelling and they like the openness of seeking. Wuthnow also sees an emerging practice-oriented spirituality that emphasizes an ongoing, constant commitment to doing the hard work of nurturing spirituality. Thus, we become what we do, and returning to spiritual practice over and over again creates habits of mind and habits of being that in time seem natural. But because spiritual practices are most often part of an open spiritual context, these habits become enlivening instead of stifling.

If all we did was to look at these three types of spirituality and how they play out in the lives of individuals over time and in various birth cohorts as they experience aging, we would have a much more complex, interesting, and authentic view of spirituality and aging than is currently available in gerontology. We would have a view that more accurately matches the complexity and importance of spirituality in the lives of most aging people.

MAJOR POINTS

This book has covered a wide variety of subjects. It represents my attempt to tie together various ideas in the vast field of spirituality and aging. If nothing else, it is an example of how the jumble of concepts and empirical evidence in the field can be put together into a meaningful mosaic. I hope this effort will serve as a starting point for those who wish to do research, teaching, and service in this field.

Much of the argument is based philosophically in an open-systems view of spirituality—what it is, how it kindles itself within human beings, how people develop their capacity for spiritual experience, how various aspects of the phenomenal world stimulate a human concern with the spiritual, how spirituality influences the development of identity and self, and how years of spiritual journeying affect an individual's ways of being in the social world—especially through lifestyles and compassionate service to others. Millions of aging people in America, perhaps a billion or more throughout the world, are aiming to live a more integrated spiritual life, one in which spirituality does not have to be reserved for one or two relatively marginal compartments of life but can flourish as a centerpiece of values and behavior.

While most of the literature views spirituality as a positive force in human life despite its difficulties and frustrations, there is a danger in an overly individualistic approach. Most people recognize the difficulty of accurately interpreting their spiritual insights and the important role that discussion and feedback can play in honing the individual's capacity for expression and discernment. In a community of spiritual peers who are each presumed to have some capacity for wisdom, it is much more difficult for spiritual insights to be converted into ego agendas. Thus, spiritual community is not only about belonging but also about support, checks and balances, and feedback along the spiritual journey.

Spirituality is an abstract, sensitizing concept that refers to a region of human experience involving awareness of being and transcending a purely personal, self-centered viewpoint. Spirituality is a subjective, existential region of experience. Spiritual experience begins with basic spirituality, an unadorned sense of being. To this is added a sense of "I" as perceiver and actor, having the capacity to experience spiritual qualities through various human avenues of experience. Spiritual experiences have identifiable qualities, such as clarity and discernment, awakening of compassion, wonder and awe, intangibility, ineffability, and they can occur through a variety of avenues: physical, sensory, consciousness/awareness, thought, intuition, transcendence. Spiritual experiences may or may not be consciously associated with or conceptually linked to the sacred or a higher power.

Spiritual experiences are related to many other aspects of spirituality, such as spiritual growth, spiritual capacity, spiritual identity and self, spiritual history, spiritual concepts and language, spiritual practice, spiritual break-through, spiritual process, and spiritual community.

Spirituality is a human capacity, which all people probably have to some extent. Developing this capacity is mysterious in that not everyone perceives or accepts the invitation to spiritual consciousness. Yet by later life, a large majority of people are in touch with and value their inner life and can identify elements of their lives that they perceive to be spiritual. This has been found in numerous studies, beginning with Clark and Anderson's (1967) wonderful ethnography of aging in middle America.[1]

Since the 1950s, the concept of spirituality as a focus of human growth and development has grown substantially in importance. Meaning is increasingly found more through an "inside-out" process of spiritual journeying, alone or in groups, and less in an "outside-in" process of learning and conforming to a religious culture. Nevertheless, most people continue to use religious ideas as resources for their spiritual journeying. In a spiritually oriented religios-ity, however, the authority is heavily vested in an inner existential process of "authenticity" and less in the authority of religious doctrines or functionar-ies. Even those who participate in a "charismatic" religious process expect the charismatic leader to kindle authentic experiences within them, to kindle their spirituality (Roof 1999).

The growing importance of spirituality is reflected by a rapidly expanding literature concerning the nature of spirituality, spiritual growth, and spiritu-ally centered lifestyles. Workshops and retreat opportunities abound, and a large proportion of the population between ages 45 and 65 is involved in small groups within which they explore their spirituality and nurture their spiritual journeys. Even within established religious denominations, such small groups have become a vital way in which people integrate spirituality into their lives. Most people believe that they are responsible for their own spiritual experi-ence and journey. Yet this popular heightening of interest in spirituality has not spread to gerontology.

Spirituality intersects with aging because spirituality increases in impor-tance as people age. This has been found in several longitudinal panel studies that followed the same individuals over time (Atchley 1999; Clark and Ander-son 1967; Fiske and Chiriboga 1990; Roof 1999). Years of experience on a spiri-tual journey usually improves a person's capacity to experience the spiritual qualities of a large array of experiences, so the spiritual consciousness of indi-viduals has a tendency to expand as they age. This occurs even in people who are not aware of being on a spiritual journey. Spirituality is a major resource for most people in coping with changes that occur as a result of aging, including "negative" changes, such as widowhood and disability, but also "positive" changes, such as retirement and grandparenthood (Atchley 2006). Spiritual experiences heavily influence values, especially the fine tuning of long-standing values, and this influence increases with age. Spirituality infuses the lives of a large proportion of older people, so spirituality is not a peripheral topic for gerontology—it is a vital context for understanding aging. Spirituality thus deserves to be a major topic in its own right within gerontology. As the baby boomers age, spirituality will be increasingly important in understanding the priorities and aspirations of aging people (Roof 1999). The goal of this book is to provide a systematic treatment of spirituality as a subject in its own right and to expand the view of spirituality within gerontology to begin to match the richness and complexity that it has in the everyday worlds of most middle-aged and older people.

IMPLICATIONS FOR INQUIRY: AVOID REINVENTING THE WHEEL

To avoid reinventing the wheel, we need to educate ourselves deeply about what has come before us. Although it is true that gerontology has not done much with questions about spirituality and aging, this does not mean that nothing exists in the historical record. I will illustrate the value of this by referring to several books that offer great potential riches to those who would study spirituality, including spirituality and aging.

William James

In 1901 and 1902, William James, Harvard professor and founding figure in American psychology, gave a series of twenty lectures that were later published under the title *The Varieties of Religious Experience: A Study in Human Nature*. In that era, *spirituality* as a term to describe direct subjective experience of the sacred was not in the vocabulary of psychology, but it is clear from the text that James was interested in spirituality, and he expressly says that he is not dealing with religious organization, doctrine, or practice. He defined "personal religion" as "the feelings, acts, and experiences of individual[s] in their solitude, so far as they apprehend themselves to stand in relation to whatever they consider the divine" (James 1905 [2005], 37). He then proceeded to probe the psychological aspects of many spiritual topics still current today:

the unseen reality of the spiritual, spirituality and health, spirituality and the self, conversion experiences, mysticism, and many others.

James achieved a remarkable clarity of conceptual and existential understanding of his subject, and I have learned a lot from him. For example, James felt that spirituality has its roots in mystical states of consciousness, which he defined as having four characteristics: ineffability (it can't be transferred or imparted to others); noetic quality (mystical states involve knowing as well as feeling); transiency (mystical states cannot be sustained long but the memory of them gives us a sense of depth and richness), and passivity (mystical states cannot be "produced"—we must be prepared to wait for them to appear). Mystical states lead us to understanding: "Our normal waking consciousness, rational consciousness as we call it, is but one special type of consciousness, whilst all about it, parted from it by the filmiest of screens, there lie potential forms of consciousness entirely different. We may go through life without suspecting their existence, but apply the requisite stimulus, and at a touch they are there in all their completeness" (ibid., 383). James makes excellent use of his own introspection and a variety of case materials and illustrates well the value of a multimethod approach.

Aldous Huxley

Aldous Huxley was a well-known novelist and highly regarded intellectual who became interested in spirituality in the 1930s and published *The Perennial Philosophy* in 1944. The book is a beautifully written and well-integrated anthology of wisdom about an underlying philosophy that can be used to understand the subjective nature of spirituality and how it plays out in various aspects of life. The enormous variety of topics covered include the relation of individual consciousness to the ground of being, the nature of the ground of being, self-knowledge, compassion, truth, grace and free will, good and evil, time and eternity, salvation and enlightenment, silence, prayer, suffering, faith, and spiritual practice. One of the major strengths of the book is that for each issue, the reader is exposed to the words used by numerous people, from a variety of religious and cultural backgrounds, whose writings have stood the test of time. The reader thus comes to a triangulated understanding of the concept at issue, an understanding that is close to what researchers call "construct validity." Huxley offers three important words of advice to those who wish to know about spirituality: detachment, charity, and humility. He is a strong advocate for the position that to study spirituality adequately, the investigator has to be willing to try contemplative methods.

Ken Wilber

Ken Wilber provides a useful perspective on the epistemology of spirituality, that is, how we come to know about this region of human experience. In his book *Eye to Eye* (2001), Wilber discusses three "eyes" (methods) through which we "see" (know). The first is the eye of our senses and technological extensions of our senses, whereby we come to know about the external world of space, time, and objects. The second is the eye of reason, through which we come to know philosophy, logic, and the mind itself. The third is the eye of contemplation, through which we come to know transcendent realities.

The process of knowing in each of these three realms has a similar structure: procedure, illumination, and confirmation. "If you do ——, then you may come to understand ——, which needs to be confirmed by ——." The procedure, the form of illumination, and the nature of confirmation is different in each of the three "eyes." Procedure is empirical in the eye of the senses, logical in the eye of reason, and meditative in the eye of contemplation. Illumination takes the form of generalization in the eye of the senses, induction in the eye of reason, and intuition in the eye of contemplation. Intersubjective agreement among peers is the root of confirmation for all three major ways of knowing. The difference lies in who one's peers are considered to be.

Wilber's central point is that each way of knowing provides valuable knowledge and that no one way of knowing can cover all subjects. Thus, to study spirituality we need sensory knowing to understand sensory spiritual experiences, intellectual knowing to see relationships among different aspects of spirituality, and contemplative knowing to understand the nature of transcendence. If gerontology is to understand spirituality, a substantial number of researchers will need to spend time learning the methods and procedures of contemplative knowing.

In the study of spirituality, there is currently a deep chasm between people who emphasize empirical and logical knowing and those who emphasize contemplative and intuitive knowing. The empiricists have little interest in, nor do they attach much credibility to, contemplative or intuitive knowing, which they see as "soft" and lacking in "precision." People who emphasize contemplative or intuitive knowing dismiss empirical and logical knowing as "overly mechanistic" and lacking in "heart." Neither side in this unfortunate conflict seems to see that they need each other. Wilber's perspective creates a bridge over this chasm, but the two sides have hardened positions that so far have prevented them from seeing its benefit.

IMPLICATIONS FOR INQUIRY: FOCUS RESEARCH ON SPIRITUALITY AS ITS OWN TOPIC

As a concept, *research* has so many possible meanings that most people cannot keep them all in mind, so they tend to think of research as referring to the types of research that predominate in their own fields. The following discussion is tedious, but I think it is important to understand in some detail the extent to which the study of spirituality has been neglected in gerontology. Think about the following types of research: experiments, surveys, field observation, records review, literature review, historical research, interpretive analysis of in-depth interviews or texts, and meta-analysis of multiple types of research. Even this list is not exhaustive. Then think about the various types of survey research: forced-choice, self-administered surveys (mail or distributed/collected); interview surveys (forced choice, open-ended, forced choice with a few open-ended); opinion surveys (mostly phone). Then think about survey design: cross-sectional slice of the population or targeted subgroup of the population, panel study of the same individuals over time, cohort sequential study of the same cohort over time (but not necessarily the same people), and key informant surveys designed to harvest the knowledge of people highly experienced in a given aspect of life. There is no one of these ways of doing research that does not have application in the study of spirituality and aging, yet by far the dominant form of research is forced-choice survey, either by mail or phone, and most of the time only a few items on spirituality are included in a much larger array of items. Sometimes the survey will be followed up with in-depth interviews of a few dozen respondents to the larger survey.

This emphasis on surveys is illustrated by an ambitious research project sponsored by the Fetzer Institute and the National Institute on Aging that resulted in a report entitled *Multidimensional Measurement of Religiousness/ Spirituality for Use in Health Research* (Fetzer Institute 2003).[2] Note that the focus was on religiousness/spirituality, as if these topics were so intertwined as to be inseparable. The project looked at questionnaire items from previous research on a wide variety of topics: daily spiritual experiences, meaning, values, beliefs, forgiveness, private religious practices, religious/spiritual coping, religious support, religious/spiritual history, commitment, organizational religiousness, and religious preference. No conceptual or theoretical background or framework was presented that would help researchers approach the issue of assessment from a deep understanding of the complex nature of the phenomena being measured.

For example, the "Daily *Spiritual* Experiences" category [emphasis added] includes items that are clearly based in a particular *religious* view—"I feel God's presence," "During worship, or at other times when connecting with God, I feel joy which lifts me out of my daily concerns," "I ask for God's help in the midst of daily activities," "I feel guided by God in the midst of daily activities," "I feel God's love for me directly," "I feel God's love for me, through others," "I desire to be closer to God or in union with Him," and "How close do you feel to God?" From many Jewish/Christian religious perspectives, this language might be an effective way of asking about the connection between religious theology and spiritual experience. But what about the 40 percent of respondents who are "unchurched" (Lindsay 2000)? What would be their response? Other items provided ambiguous answers about spirituality: "I find strength in my religion or spirituality" and "I find comfort in my religion or spirituality." If someone says "every day" to these questions, is their response about religion or about spirituality? There is no way to tell. Similar conceptual problems exist in all the areas covered by the report.

Based on the conceptual/theoretical framework provided in Chapter 2 of this volume, some items from the Fetzer report seem to qualify as assessments of spirituality: "I experience a connection to all of life," "I feel deep inner peace or harmony," "I am spiritually touched by the beauty of [nature]" (The actual word was *creation,* a religiously loaded word), and "I feel a selfless caring for others." So it does seem possible to ask sensible, inclusive questions about spiritual experience. Note that to make this determination, to have this discernment, I used criteria from my conceptual/theoretical framework about spirituality.

To increase the chances that questions on religion and spirituality might be included in large-scale surveys, the Fetzer/NIA working group developed a 38-item "Brief Multidimensional Measure of Religiousness/Spirituality." Of these items, 28 clearly dealt with religion, 6 were clearly about spirituality, and 4 were ambiguous. Many of the religion questions were cast in Jewish/Christian language.

The Fetzer report no doubt was done by people who worked hard and took their jobs seriously. The report's flaws reflect accurately the widespread oversimplification of and confusion about spirituality that is imbedded in gerontology—and most other social sciences, for that matter. The Fetzer report illustrates the "state of the art" concerning measurement or assessment of individual spirituality. I do not mean to be any more critical of the Fetzer/NIA working group than I would be of the groups that created all of the other existing measures that indiscriminately mix religion and spirituality and thus continue to confuse the issue.

To invite more conversation on this issue by survey researchers, I offer my *Spirituality Inventory* in Appendix A. Its 85 items have been written with an eye not only for content but also for wording that is inclusive. These items have been pretested on a small sample of older adults and generally can be answered by most respondents, but much study and refinement remains to be done to identify the psychometric properties of the inventory.

For qualitative researchers, Appendix B consists of my open-ended Questions for Reflection and Spiritual Self-Assessment, which can be adapted for use as an interview guide. In keeping with my theoretical framework, these questions are designed to provide feedback to individuals about their spiritual journey. Chapter 6 discussed the possible uses of these questions by practitioners who wish to do spiritual assessment.

Much of the literature on spirituality is based on variants of a single question: "To what extent do you consider yourself a spiritual person?" While answers to this question are certainly of interest, they leave many more questions begging to be asked. It is difficult to avoid the conclusion that gerontology as a field does not really want to know much about spirituality and does not consider it very important, yet spirituality shows up in the top tier of personal values of a large majority of elders.

To advance our understanding of spirituality and aging, we do not need more research projects; we need more research programs. Research projects are designed to study limited topics carefully and serve knowledge building in an incremental way. Research programs can study a subject with many coordinated research projects, which can employ a variety of perspectives and methods. The expanded view of spirituality and aging in this book cries out for research programs.

IMPLICATIONS FOR GERONTOLOGY EDUCATION

If we want to include spirituality in research and practice in gerontology we have to begin to teach in depth about spirituality and aging. As it stands now, introductory students rarely get more than a few minutes' discussion of spirituality, if that. Religion and spirituality are often lumped together, with religion getting the bulk of the attention. Few people specialize in the study of spirituality, and most gerontology professors are probably intimidated by the prospect of teaching about something they do not have in-depth knowledge of. I hope that this book will help them be more comfortable teaching about spirituality as a subject in its own right.

Spirituality should be included in any gerontology education program that aspires to teach a holistic perspective. For today's students, the compartmentalized separation of courses may be outdated. What may be more effective is to begin with research and practice topics and show how holistic and multidisciplinary perspectives can lead to more effective research and practice. Thus, we could consider spirituality as an important factor relevant to lifestyle choices, adaptation to life events, intergenerational relationships, and so on. If we were to look, we might find this to be true. The limited evidence we have suggests that it is.

The implications of the entry of the baby boomers into the older population are high on many lists of considerations concerning program planning. In Roof's (1999) large panel study of boomers, most respondents felt that spirituality—an inner path or journey—was a central concern, whether the journey took place in a religious context or not. Seventy-three percent of Roof's respondents said they were significantly spiritual. They felt that they were responsible for coming to their own understanding of issues about meaning and faith. Religion was judged on the basis of what it could contribute to that understanding. Most felt quite free to mix and match ideas and practices from a variety of spiritual and religious traditions to form their own unique approach to spirituality. Most were also involved in small groups of fellow seekers who supported and nurtured one another's spiritual journey. Given that the upcoming older population is using open-systems approaches to spirituality, and religious authority is less crucial, understanding spirituality will become even more important for gerontology.

An open-systems approach presumes that the system is evolving based on experience with using it. Thus, the system for dealing with the spiritual journey and openness about precisely where the journey will lead can be expected to supplant former views of spirituality oriented around conformity and security. Systems seldom remain in equilibrium long enough to identify what one would conform to. Instead, a premium is placed on being able to respond effectively to whatever happens. Part of today's spiritual journeys requires having faith in the system's direction of movement rather than in a specific outcome. This fits right in with a practice of dwelling in the questions rather than fixating on today's answers. To deal with tomorrow's spirituality, students and their teachers will do well to try theories built around open-feedback systems. At several points in the book, I have used examples from continuity theory, which is an example of an open-feedback-systems theory.

An open-feedback-systems approach to spirituality has two important advantages: flexibility and less potential for divisiveness. Because the system is in a constant state of feedback, it remains flexible. Because an open-systems approach to spirituality is rooted in individually created personal constructs, people can see their viewpoint in the system, and there is less incentive to try to annihilate other viewpoints.

A major disadvantage to systems theory is that it does not offer specific, stable solutions "once and for all." Some people need a "once and for all" level of certainty, and they are unlikely to be served by an open-feedback-systems approach to spirituality. Another disadvantage is that such approaches do not produce "The Seven Habits of Highly Spiritual People." Systems approaches advocate for systems approaches, not a particular system or recipe. *You* find out if *your system* works *for you* by observing it in action.

Students will be more attracted to the study of spirituality and aging if they are allowed to work on their own spiritual process at the same time. If they are encouraged to engage the same questions the research participants are responding to, the students have a greater potential to become better researchers or practitioners. To the extent that students experience their own spirituality, they may come to better appreciate the role spirituality plays for elders. A nonreligious language of spirituality may help by allowing students to discuss spirituality without being drawn into discussions of differences in theology or religious doctrine.

SPIRITUALITY AND AGING FOR PRACTITIONERS

For people who work directly with aging people a big question is, Who is the client? Is it the stereotyped feeble older person who has no life and is lonely? Or is it a vitally involved person on a spiritual journey despite the inconveniences and losses that can come with age? Or is it another spiritual being just like them but in a different human form? George Fox, a founder of Quakerism, said we should go joyfully about the world, answering that of God in everyone. Fox's point was to respond to the basic spirituality of each person and not the personality or social background. At the level of basic spirituality, what is there to get into conflict about or to object to? What would happen if we learned to tune into the basic spirituality of the people being served? To tune into the spirituality of those being served, would we need to tune into our own? Would trying to tune into the basic spirituality of another person help us tune into our own?

The expanded view of spirituality presented in this book provides a framework for learning important things about many of the people we work with. There are few things more important to many aging people than their intentions for their own spiritual journey. But we cannot assume that we know anything about those intentions or that we have even a basic outline of how they see that journey. We have to wait for them to tell us in their own time and in their own way. Some will tell us in words, others in body language, others in the art they make, others through the music they sing. How does a person reveal his or her basic spirituality? It can done in any of a hundred ways. To see it, we must create a safe place, one in which aging persons can express themselves.

Earlier I wrote that to study spirituality, researchers benefit from being able to use their own spiritual capacities and perspectives. So it is with serving the spirituality of clients. *How Can I Help?* (Ram Dass and Gorman 1995) is the best resource I have seen on how to help from a spiritually awakened place. The authors begin with the notion that we all have an impulse to care when faced with others in need. Whether we translate that impulse into action depends on how we deal with barriers to the natural expression of caring. Spiritually grounded caring comes from compassion, not pity.

> Compassion and pity are very different. Whereas compassion reflects the yearning of the heart to merge and take on some of the suffering, pity is a controlled set of thoughts designed to assure separateness. Compassion is the spontaneous response of love; pity, the involuntary reflex of fear. (Ibid., 62)

> ⚭

> Who *are* we to ourselves and to one another?—it will all come down to that. *Will we look within?* Can we see that to be of most service to others we must face our own doubts, needs, and resistances? (Ibid., 15)

To see situations clearly and dispassionately, we benefit from learning to see things from nonpersonal consciousness, or *witness consciousness,* as Ram Dass and Gorman label it.

Witnessing is dispassionate. It's not committed to one result or another; it's open to everything. Because it has . . . no axe to grind, it is more able to see truth. As the Tao Te Ching says, "The truth awaits for eyes unclouded by longing." The Witness, however, is not passive, complacent, or indifferent. Indeed, while it's not attached to a particular outcome, its presence turns out to bring about change. As we bring *what is* into the light of clear awareness, we begin to see that the universe is providing us with abundant clues to the nature of the suffering before us, what is being asked, what fears have been inhibiting us, and, finally, *what might really help*. All we have to do is listen—really listen. (Ibid., 68–69)

Thus, commitment to objectivity turns out to be a spiritual practice that is essential to doing effective service.

> Light from within, that's our illumination.
> To dwell in silent peace, that's our meditation.
> To see the passing world, with clearness and compassion.
> And when we clearly see, we are drawn to BE love and to serve.
>
> Atchley (1996)

A CHALLENGE

Some may be drawn to the study of spirituality and aging for purely intellectual or pragmatic reasons—well and good. I suspect more will be drawn to this subject because it also has appeal to them from within themselves and from their experiences of aging individuals. When I was interviewing older people early in my career, I encountered many sages, people who seemed to possess wisdom born of a life experience that had been *reflected upon*. They had a vitality and presence that I admired. "I want to be like that when I'm old," I thought. Today, I *am* like that. This did not happen by accident. I kept their example as a guide for the direction I wanted to take, and in my own way and with my own system I have learned much of what I needed to learn and developed the habits I needed to develop. I also had to persist through times of confusion and doubt. Along the way I benefited greatly from persistent study, many excellent teachers, earnest practice, and several supportive spiritual communities.

I can attest to the value of being on an intentional spiritual journey whose purpose is to find within oneself the nonpersonal consciousness needed to approach objectivity. I can also attest that this "road less traveled" is not an easy one. There is much prejudice against "the spiritual" within the scientific and academic communities. The inner journey itself is filled with paradoxes. But this inner journey, which thrives on ideas tested by experience, can become a process worthy of faith.

My challenge to you is to engage the possibilities of spirituality and aging. I am not suggesting that you *believe* anything I have said. I am challenging you try these ideas out, to use the framework given here and see what happens. Contribute your feedback. Revise and improve. Junk this framework and make a better one of your own. But please do not abandon the important subject of spirituality and aging.

Spirituality Inventory

Please place a check mark by the word(s) that best describes your response to the statement or question.

   1. The word *spiritual* has meaning for me.

   _____ Strongly agree

   _____ Agree

   _____ Disagree

   _____ Strongly disagree

   2. Do you consider yourself spiritual?

   _____ Strongly agree

   _____ Agree

   _____ Disagree

   _____ Strongly disagree

   3. Do you consider yourself spiritual?

   _____ Always

   _____ Often

   _____ Sometimes

   _____ Seldom

   _____ Never

4. I am a person who has spiritual experiences.

____ Strongly agree

____ Agree

____ Disagree

____ Strongly disagree

5. My spiritual experiences include direct experiences of a higher power.

____ Strongly agree

____ Agree

____ Disagree

____ Strongly disagree

6. I am on a spiritual journey.

____ Strongly agree

____ Agree

____ Disagree

____ Strongly disagree

If you are on a spiritual journey, how long have you been on it? ____ Years

What age were you when your journey began? ____ Years

7. My spiritual journey has been marked by ups and downs.

____ Strongly agree

____ Agree

____ Disagree

____ Strongly disagree

8. To what extent do you consider yourself a spiritual person?

_____ Very spiritual

_____ Moderately spiritual

_____ Slightly spiritual

_____ Slightly nonspiritual

_____ Moderately nonspiritual

_____ Very nonspiritual

9. To what extent do you consider yourself a religious person?

_____ Very religious

_____ Moderately religious

_____ Slightly religious

_____ Slightly nonreligious

_____ Moderately nonreligious

_____ Very nonreligious

10. I participate in an organized spiritual community.

_____ Often

_____ Sometimes

_____ Seldom

_____ Never

11. I organize my life around participation in my spiritual community.

_____ Often

_____ Sometimes

_____ Seldom

_____ Never

12. I can count on my spiritual community for help.

____ Strongly agree

____ Agree

____ Disagree

____ Strongly disagree

13. I can count on my spiritual community for guidance.

____ Strongly agree

____ Agree

____ Disagree

____ Strongly disagree

14. On average, how many hours a week do you spend doing unpaid work for your spiritual community? ____ Hours

15. I can count on my spiritual community for care.

____ Strongly agree

____ Agree

____ Disagree

____ Strongly disagree

16. I sometimes find my spiritual community too critical.

____ Strongly agree

____ Agree

____ Disagree

____ Strongly disagree

17. I sometimes find my spiritual community too demanding.

____ Strongly agree

____ Agree

____ Disagree

____ Strongly disagree

18. I have a philosophy of life that helps me understand my spiritual experiences.

____ Strongly agree

____ Agree

____ Disagree

____ Strongly disagree

19. I am a spiritual being having a human journey.

____ Strongly agree

____ Agree

____ Disagree

____ Strongly disagree

20. Spirituality is an important part of who I am.

____ Strongly agree

____ Agree

____ Disagree

____ Strongly disagree

21. I try to bring my spiritual perspective into my [check all that apply]:

____ lifestyle

____ family life

____ work

____ community participation

____ religious participation

22. An important part of the meaning of life for me comes from my spiritual experiences.

____ Strongly agree

____ Agree

____ Disagree

____ Strongly disagree

23. My spiritual perspective serves me well in most of my life.

____ Strongly agree

____ Agree

____ Disagree

____ Strongly disagree

24. I have confidence and trust in my way of understanding and acting on my spiritual experiences.

____ Strongly agree

____ Agree

____ Disagree

____ Strongly disagree

25. I have confidence and trust in my way of understanding and acting on my spiritual experiences.

____ Always

____ Often

____ Sometimes

____ Seldom

____ Never

26. I have had spiritual experiences that changed my life.

____ Strongly agree

____ Agree

____ Disagree

____ Strongly disagree

If so, about how many times? ____ Events

27. My spirituality helps me deal with stressful situations.

____ Strongly agree

____ Agree

____ Disagree

____ Strongly disagree

28. There is a part of me that seems eternal.

____ Strongly agree

____ Agree

____ Disagree

____ Strongly disagree

29. To nurture my spiritual life, I [check all that apply]:

____ pray

____ meditate

____ read articles and books about spiritual topics

____ listen to audio or watch video presentations about spiritual topics

____ contemplate spiritual issues

____ engage in "good works"

____ participate in movement disciplines such as yoga or labyrinth walking

____ participate in spiritual discussions

____ participate in spiritual workshops or retreats

____ engage in private spiritual devotions

____ attend religious services

In all, I devote about ____ hours a week to these activities.

30. I participate in spiritually oriented small groups.

____ Yes, often

____ Yes, occasionally

____ No

31. I read and ponder articles and books about spiritual topics.

____ Many times each day

____ Every day

____ Most days

____ Some days

____ Seldom

____ Never

32. I read spiritually stimulating texts.

_____ Many times each day

_____ Every day

_____ Most days

_____ Some days

_____ Seldom

_____ Never

33. I pray alone.

_____ Many times each day

_____ Every day

_____ Most days

_____ Some days

_____ Seldom

_____ Never

34. I meditate.

_____ Many times each day

_____ Every day

_____ Most days

_____ Some days

_____ Seldom

_____ Never

35. I feel motivated to help reduce pain and suffering in the world.

_____ Always

_____ Often

_____ Sometimes

_____ Seldom

_____ Never

36. I feel motivated to help reduce pain and suffering in the world.

_____ Strongly agree

_____ Agree

_____ Disagree

_____ Strongly disagree

37. I am spiritually touched by nature's wonders.

_____ Strongly agree

_____ Agree

_____ Disagree

_____ Strongly disagree

38. I feel deep inner peace and stillness.

_____ Always

_____ Often

_____ Sometimes

_____ Seldom

_____ Never

39. My spiritual life brings me strength.

____ Often

____ Sometimes

____ Seldom

____ Never

40. My spiritual life brings me comfort.

____ Often

____ Sometimes

____ Seldom

____ Never

41. My spiritual life brings me uncertainty.

____ Often

____ Sometimes

____ Seldom

____ Never

42. My spiritual life brings me confusion.

____ Often

____ Sometimes

____ Seldom

____ Never

43. I feel a sacred presence.

____ Always

____ Often

____ Sometimes

____ Seldom

____ Never

44. I experience a connection with all of life.

____ Always

____ Often

____ Sometimes

____ Seldom

____ Never

45. My spiritual worldview gives meaning to life's ups and downs.

____ Strongly agree

____ Agree

____ Disagree

____ Strongly disagree

46. Without a sense of spirituality, my daily life would have less meaning.

____ Strongly agree

____ Agree

____ Disagree

____ Strongly disagree

47. When I feel disconnected from my spirituality, my sense of purpose is less clear.

_____ Strongly agree

_____ Agree

_____ Disagree

_____ Strongly disagree

48. I feel that I am part of something much greater than my personal self.

_____ Always

_____ Often

_____ Sometimes

_____ Seldom

_____ Never

49. What I choose to do in my daily life is important to me spiritually.

_____ Strongly agree

_____ Agree

Disagree

_____ Strongly disagree

50. My spirituality helps me deal with troubling or confusing events.

_____ Strongly agree

_____ Agree

_____ Disagree

_____ Strongly disagree

51. My experience of spirituality adds meaning to my everyday life.

_____ Strongly agree

_____ Agree

_____ Disagree

_____ Strongly disagree

52. For me, forgiving myself and others is an important spiritual practice.

_____ Strongly agree

_____ Agree

_____ Disagree

_____ Strongly disagree

53. Commitment to spiritual concerns is one of my most important personal values.

_____ Strongly agree

_____ Agree

_____ Disagree

_____ Strongly disagree

54. I am strongly committed to my spiritual journey.

_____ Strongly agree

_____ Agree

_____ Disagree

_____ Strongly disagree

55. Paying attention to my spiritual journey is important to me.

____ Strongly agree

____ Agree

____ Disagree

____ Strongly disagree

56. Nurturing my spiritual journey is important to me.

____ Strongly agree

____ Agree

____ Disagree

____ Strongly disagree

57. I am confident concerning what I believe about spirituality.

____ Strongly agree

____ Agree

____ Disagree

____ Strongly disagree

58. Spirituality is a quality that can be part of *any* life experience.

____ Strongly agree

____ Agree

____ Disagree

____ Strongly disagree

59. Spirituality is a different type of experience, easily distinguished from other types of experience.

____ Strongly agree

____ Agree

____ Disagree

____ Strongly disagree

60. For me, spiritual experiences occur through my [check all that apply]:

____ senses

____ bodily sensations

____ emotions

____ thoughts

____ awareness

____ transcendence

61. Over the years, my capacity to experience spirituality has grown.

____ Strongly agree

____ Agree

____ Disagree

____ Strongly disagree

62. I experience a presence of the supreme being.

____ Strongly agree

____ Agree

____ Disagree

____ Strongly disagree

63. My capacity for spiritual experience has become more effective over the years.

____ Strongly agree

____ Agree

____ Disagree

____ Strongly disagree

64. Spirituality is an important part of my life story.

____ Strongly agree

____ Agree

____ Disagree

____ Strongly disagree

65. I have confidence in my ways of experiencing spirituality.

____ Always

____ Often

____ Sometimes

____ Seldom

____ Never

66. I have confidence in my ways of acting on my spiritual insights.

____ Always

____ Often

____ Sometimes

____ Seldom

____ Never

67. I have doubts about my ways of dealing with my spirituality.

____ Always

____ Often

____ Sometimes

____ Seldom

____ Never

68. My spiritual process is open to new types of experience.

____ Strongly agree

____ Agree

____ Disagree

____ Strongly disagree

69. My spiritual life causes me suffering.

____ Often

____ Sometimes

____ Seldom

____ Never

70. For me, there could be no spirituality without my religion.

____ Strongly agree

____ Agree

____ Disagree

____ Strongly disagree

71. Spirituality and religion are the same thing to me.

_____ Strongly agree

_____ Agree

_____ Disagree

_____ Strongly disagree

72. My spirituality rests firmly in religious ideas and practices.

_____ Strongly agree

_____ Agree

_____ Disagree

_____ Strongly disagree

73. My religious community is my main spiritual community.

_____ Strongly agree

_____ Agree

_____ Disagree

_____ Strongly disagree

74. Religious rituals are an important type of spiritual experience for me.

_____ Strongly agree

_____ Agree

_____ Disagree

_____ Strongly disagree

75. My spirituality brings me joy and appreciation.

_____ Strongly agree

_____ Agree

_____ Disagree

_____ Strongly disagree

76. My spirituality brings me joy and appreciation.

_____ Always

_____ Often

_____ Sometimes

_____ Seldom

_____ Never

77. My spiritual experiences have had a strong influence on what I believe.

_____ Strongly agree

_____ Agree

_____ Disagree

_____ Strongly disagree

78. My spirituality has a strong influence on my relationships with others.

_____ Strongly agree

_____ Agree

_____ Disagree

_____ Strongly disagree

79. My spirituality has a strong influence on my relationships with others.

____ Always

____ Often

____ Sometimes

____ Seldom

____ Never

80. When I pay attention to spirituality, life seems to go better for me.

____ Strongly agree

____ Agree

____ Disagree

____ Strongly disagree

81. When I pay attention to spirituality, life seems to go better for me.

____ Always

____ Often

____ Sometimes

____ Seldom

____ Never

82. I feel alienated from my spirituality.

____ Always

____ Often

____ Sometimes

____ Seldom

____ Never

83. My spirituality conflicts with my personal desires and fears.

_____ Always

_____ Often

_____ Sometimes

_____ Seldom

_____ Never

84. My spiritual perspective helps me see my world more clearly.

_____ Strongly agree

_____ Agree

_____ Disagree

_____ Strongly disagree

85. I participate in more than one spiritual community.

_____ Yes   How many in all? _____

_____ No

Questions for Reflection and Spiritual Self-Assessment

I beg you . . . to have patience with everything unresolved
in your heart and try to love the questions themselves as
if they were locked rooms or books written in a very for-
eign language. Don't search for the answers, which could
not be given to you now, because you would not be able
to live them. And the point is to live everything. Live the
questions now. Perhaps then someday far in the future
you will gradually, without ever noticing it, live your way
into the answer.   —*Rainer Maria Rilke*

The questions that follow are not a test. Instead, they are invitations to self-reflection. Whether one has a clear answer, a murky answer, or no answer is as it is. The questions are couched in the first person to indicate that they are posed to the reader, and the answers that matter most are answers coming from the reader's own experience. Most of the questions are enduring questions, and responses to them probably evolve over time. Don't be discouraged if answers don't appear immediately. Return often to the questions, with openness and honesty, and see what happens. It may also be helpful to explore questions of particular interest with a group of spiritual friends that meets periodically for this purpose.

What is my spiritual nature?

What is my essential nature? Is there an eternal part of me? What is my source? Where does my consciousness/awareness come from? If there is "that of God" or "the Absolute" in me, how do I experience this aspect?

⁂

What is spirituality? Is there a part of my experience that I would label "spiritual?" What qualifies an experience to be called "spiritual"? Is spirituality a capacity for a certain *type* of experience? How do spiritual experiences interact with other experiences I have? Is spiritual experience something separate or is it a *quality* that can accompany all experiences? or can it be both?

⊕

Is there a part of me that is especially sensitive to spiritual experiences? Can the mind have a spiritual experience? the body? How are emotions related to spiritual experience? Is there something in me beyond body and mind?

⊕

Do I have a spiritual center? If so, is it in the body, in consciousness, in the mind, in all three, or beyond all of these, or all of the above? Is there more to the mind than thought? Are emotions manifested through the body?

⊕

Is spirituality a *quality* of being that underlies all other experience? (Compare a computer program that runs in the background.) If so, how do I know about this aspect of spirituality? If spirituality is a quality of being, are there different grades or shades or levels of it?

⊕

How do I *know* these things?

What does it mean to grow spiritually?

Do I aspire to grow spiritually? If so, what supports this aspiration? What interferes? Does growing spiritually occur in stages or cycles, is it continuous, or both?

⊕

Does the capacity for spiritual experience evolve? If so, what stimulates this evolution? What are "spiritual practices," and how do they relate to spiritual capacities and experiences? Is there a difference between awakening and enlightenment? Is there an end point to spiritual evolution? If so, what is it?

⊕

What happens when I die? Who dies? Is death a spiritual transition? If so, a transition from what to what?

⊕

How does my "story"—my version of my biography or personal history—relate to growing spiritually? How does my personality affect spirituality? How do social biography and social relationships affect spirituality? Who is the doer?

⊕

Is God involved in my spiritual evolution?*

Do I have direct experiences of something I call God? If so, how does God appear to me? What is God's nature? Does God act? If so, how? Does God have will? Is God's will involved in my spiritual evolution? What is will?

Do I have confidence and trust in my spiritual process?

Does my experience lead me to confidence and trust in my ways of seeing my spiritual nature and that of my world and acting on the perceptions rooted in these ways of seeing? How do I deal with experiences that cast doubt on these ways of seeing spiritually? Does my process allow me to incorporate new experiences into my ways of seeing? Is my spirituality a resource for coping with suffering? Does my spiritual process lead to joy and appreciation?

How does my spirituality manifest itself in the world?

How do spirituality and growing spiritually relate to organized religion, religious culture, or religious behavior? Are my spirituality and religion synonymous, separate, or somewhere in between? Does spiritual experience relate to sacred texts, religious doctrines, or religious rituals? If so, how?

⁂

How does spirituality influence what I believe? How does spirituality influence my choices of goals and the priorities I set among these goals? How does spirituality influence my behavior? Does spirituality influence my preferences concerning activities, lifestyles, and human relationships? How can I manifest my spirituality in my work? in my community? in my lifestyle?

⁂

Is there a spiritual aspect of relationships? Can a couple grow spiritually?

⁂

Can spirituality manifest in groups? Can a group grow spiritually?
Can spirituality affect culture? Can culture affect spirituality? If so, how?

---

* *God* is a word used to refer to many concepts of the supreme being. Some concepts picture God as a person-like being who thinks, has motives, goals, and aims, has a voice, and speaks to lesser beings. Other concepts view God as a great oneness, a being that includes all time and space and matter and antimatter and good and evil, a being that our dualistic minds cannot understand but that we can know through intuition. Still other concepts see God as most clearly visible in the natural world. For my spiritual evolution, is it necessary to reconcile differing views of God or is it necessary for me only to become clear about my experiences of God (possibly including the experience that God does not exist) and what these experiences imply for my spiritual evolution?

Do I envision a life undivided from my spiritual being?

What separates or divides me from my sense of spiritual being? Does it have to be this way? What could I do to remain rooted in my being as I go through all the doing that is needed in life? Does my spiritual being give me a vantage point from which to discern clearly?

✤

Can my ego and my spiritual being co-exist? If so, how?

Notes

PREFACE

1. Participants in the Omega Institute think tank met for a week at the Omega campus in Rhinebeck, New York. Participants included Ram Dass, Zalman Schachter-Shalomi, Carter Williams, Thomas Cole, Robert Atchley, H. R. Moody, Eve Ilsen, Drew Leder, Carole Segrave, Connie Goldman, and several Omega program planning staff persons. The goal of the think tank was to explore what types of educational program might be good next steps. As a result of this experience, I developed a weeklong workshop, "Spiritual Growth in Middle and Later Life," which I offered with cofacilitators Sheila Atchley and H. R. Moody in the summer of 1996. Planning and offering this workshop gave me important insights into how best to discuss this material.

INTRODUCTION: SETTING THE STAGE

1. For a listing of more-detailed questions subsumed under these general categories, see Appendix B.

2. Martin Heidegger (1966) used the term *region* to refer to a place we go in awareness when we leave the world of discursive, calculative thinking. A region is "the trackless and radiant core of Being." Thus, the spiritual region is more than a mere area; it is suffused by what Heidegger called "holy openness."

3. Lindsay (2000) found that the proportion of adults who reported being "unchurched" hovered between 40 and 45 percent over the period from 1978 to 1998, which suggests long-term stability in this factor.

4. For a discussion of the processes through which this occurred, see Robert Wuthnow (1998), chap. 2.

5. The *Bhagavad Gita*, which was written down several thousand years ago in India, is probably the earliest statement of this principle. For an excellent translation of this work, see Prabhavananda and Isherwood (1944). This idea is present in variants of the major faith traditions. It can be traced through the European literature on mysticism from the Middle Ages.

6. Abraham Maslow's *Toward a Psychology of Being* (1968) was probably the most influential statement of this point of view.

7. This is not to imply that members of the clergy cannot inspire direct, independent, and authentic spiritual experience. Many certainly do. In fact, some of the richest discussions of how to connect directly with the sacred can be found in published sermons. Meister Eckhart is a prime example. However, when religious culture teaches that spiritual connection *requires* mediation by the clergy, then I think damage can be done to the human spirit. For example, Valerie grew up Catholic, and when she was about 9 she started asking Jesus to talk to her, and she was somewhat surprised when He actually did. She heard a voice that was not her own. When she told her Catholic school teachers about this experience, the response was, "You can't possibly have talked with Jesus. He has lots more important things to do than to talk to the likes of you. That's what priests are for."

8. For a discussion of Blumer's perspective, see Turner (1991, 403).

9. The *American Heritage Dictionary* (2006) defines rumination as "the act of pondering; meditation." This is a perfect definition for my purposes; it is just what I intend. Unfortunately, the *Diagnostic Manual of Mental Disorders* (DSM-IV) lists rumination as an eating disorder. What's a writer to do? I decided I should not avoid ordinary language because some profession or academic specialty has developed a technical meaning for these same words that conflict or sometimes contradict dictionary definitions.

10. I believe both Huxley and Tillich developed this concept of ground following the influence of Martin Heidegger and Meister Eckhart. Eckhart's idea was that we needed a larger concept of a transcendent God, one that stood as the *ground* for the manifest God, with the manifest God as figure and the transcendent God as ground.

1. THE NATURE OF SPIRITUAL EXPERIENCE

1. I use the term *ground of being* to refer to that which is the supreme context for all other being. Others use *God, Allah, Yahweh, the Absolute,* and a host of other terms. Some concepts picture the supreme being as a personlike being who thinks, has motives, goals, and aims, has a voice, and speaks to lesser beings. Other concepts see the supreme being as a great oneness, a being that includes all time and space and matter and antimatter and good and evil, a being that our dualistic human minds cannot understand but that we can know through intuitive experience. Still other concepts envision the supreme being as embodied in nature. To study spirituality, it is not necessary to reconcile differing views about the nature or existence of a supreme being; it is necessary only to understand how each individual experiences and answers the question of the supreme being and how these experiences relate to spiritual experiences. (For more on such concepts, see Zinnbauer et al. 1997.)

2. Heidegger (1966) discussed a relationship between transcendent consciousness and thought. He contrasted calculative thinking with contemplative thinking by saying that the former is done by conventional consciousness whereas the latter

occurs in a higher level of consciousness, where it was possible to think in terms of regions with fuzzy boundaries.

2. SPIRITUAL DEVELOPMENT

1. Although the book was co-authored by Moody and Carroll, Moody conducted the research, the main theoretical ideas are Moody's, and many of the personal examples in the book are from Moody's personal experience.

3. SPIRITUALITY, SPIRITUAL SELF, AND SPIRITUAL IDENTITY

1. For more on Mead, Cooley, and other aspects of these concepts, see Turner (1991).

2. Carl Jung developed a complex and dynamic psychology that goes well beyond the scope of this chapter. Here I deal with only his notion of the "shadow self."

3. For more on the self system in later life, see Atchley (1999), chap. 2.

5. TRANSPERSONAL SOCIOLOGY AND SERVING FROM SPIRIT

1. To the best of my knowledge, the term *transpersonal sociology* was first used by Ken Wilber in *A Sociable God* (1983), which was mainly about religion. Wilber used the term to indicate a new type of possibility for religions created by people who had been transformed by transpersonal psychology. The term has been little used since then, and almost never by sociologists. Nevertheless, I believe it is time to offer a more fleshed-out statement of some principles we might expect to find useful in looking at spirituality as it plays out in community.

2. The Quakers are an example of a spiritual culture following transpersonal principles that has been successfully in operation for more than three hundred years. In contemporary culture, many cohousing communities are also attempting to live by principles of transpersonal sociology.

3. For examples of resource material taking a transpersonal sociological view of organizational leadership, see Gilley (1997) and Dreher (1996).

6. CONTINUITY, SPIRITUAL GROWTH, AND COPING IN LATER ADULTHOOD

1. The concept of integrity used by Erikson, Erikson, and Kivnick (1986) differed considerably from the concept of ego integrity used by Erikson (1955) in his earlier work. Ego integrity is a much more self-centered concept than the idea of integrity as a holistic and positive integrating force balancing the negative forces of chaos and despair.

7. SPIRITUAL BELIEFS AND PRACTICES AND THE EXPERIENCE OF TIME AND AGING

1. Habituation is a process of selectively ignoring sensory stimuli to reduce the amount of material that has to be processed by perception. Habituation is a necessary skill that allows infants to simplify sensory chaos to the point that it can be organized into perceptions. Overhabituation oversimplifies information coming from the environment to the point that nothing new seems to be happening. (See Kastenbaum 1993.)

8. SPIRITUALITY AND THE EXPERIENCE OF DYING AND DEATH

1. Unless otherwise noted, all examples are taken from my interviews and observations.

2. See Kastenbaum (2004) for a fascinating and thought-provoking discussion of the many aspects of how dying and death are thought about in American culture. Kastenbaum's book is clear evidence that even our brightest minds are humbled by the mystery that is death.

CONCLUSION

1. Interestingly, within gerontology, anthropology seems to have preserved its ties to the humanities to a much greater extent than have sociology or psychology. This is probably connected to the predominant research methods in the respective fields, because anthropologists still tend to learn through intensive open-ended interviews whereas other social scientists pursue knowledge mainly through large-scale structured sample surveys, with their relatively rigid protocols and mathematically abstracted analyses.

2. On the one hand, the Fetzer/NIA effort could be praised for making an effort to bring some precision to the study of religion, spirituality, and aging. On the other hand, by starting with flawed questions from earlier research, failing to develop an underlying theoretical/conceptual framework for discerning questions, and relying too much on quantitative, mathematical methods of winnowing, the results were fatally flawed. The results also indicate the difficulties of doing research in such politically charged areas as spirituality and religion.

References

Achenbaum, W. Andrew. 1997. *The wisdom of age: An historian's perspective.* Distinguished Lecture Series. Chapel Hill: Univ. of North Carolina Institute on Aging.

Achenbaum, W. Andrew, and Lucinda Orwoll. 1991. Becoming wise. *International Journal of Aging and Adult Development* 32: 21–39.

Agnes, Michael, ed. 2002. *Webster's New World college dictionary,* 4th ed. New York: Wiley.

American heritage dictionary of the English language, 4th ed. Boston: Houghton Mifflin, 2006.

Anon. [Fourteenth century] 2004. *The cloud of unknowing.* Ed. William Johnston. New York: HarperCollins.

Ardelt, Monika. 2003. Empirical assessment of a three-dimensional wisdom scale. *Research on Aging* 25 (3): 275–324.

Atchley, Bob [Robert C.]. 1996. *The Journey.* Original song and lyrics.

Atchley, Robert C. 1993. Spiritual development and wisdom: A Vedantic perspective. In *Encyclopedia of adult development,* ed. R. Kastenbaum, 479–83. Phoenix, AZ: Oryx Press.

———. 1997a. Everyday mysticism: Spiritual development in later life. *Journal of Adult Development* 4 (2): 123–34.

———. 1997b. *Social forces and aging,* 8th ed. Belmont, CA: Wadsworth.

———. 1999. *Continuity and adaptation in aging: Creating positive experiences.* Baltimore: Johns Hopkins Univ. Press.

———. 2000. Spirituality. In *Handbook of the humanities and aging,* ed. T. R. Cole, R. E. Ray, and R. Kastenbaum, 2nd ed., 324–41. New York: Springer.

———. 2001. The influence of spiritual beliefs and practices on the relation between time and aging. In *Aging and the meaning of time,* ed. S. H. McFadden and R. C. Atchley, 157–76. New York: Springer.

———. 2003. Becoming a spiritual elder. In *Aging, spirituality, and religion: A handbook,* ed. M. A. Kimble and S. H. McFadden, 2: 33–46. Minneapolis: Fortress Press.

———. 2005. The path of service in later adulthood. Paper presented to the Annual Meeting of the American Society on Aging. Philadelphia, March 12.

———. 2006. Continuity, spiritual growth, and coping in later adulthood. *Journal of Religion, Spirituality, and Aging* 18 (2–3): 19–29.

Atchley, Robert C., and Amanda S. Barusch. 2004. *Social forces and aging*, 10th ed. Belmont, CA: Wadsworth.

Baltes, Paul B. 1993. The aging mind: Potential and limits. *Gerontologist* 33: 580–94.

Baltes, Paul B., and Jacqui Smith. 1990. Toward a psychology of wisdom and its ontogenesis. In *Wisdom: Its nature, origins, and development*, ed. R. J. Sternberg, 87–120. Cambridge: Cambridge Univ. Press.

Baltes, Paul B., and Ursula M. Staudinger. 2000. Wisdom: A metaheuristic (pragmatic) to orchestrate mind and virtue toward excellence. *American Psychologist* 55: 122–36.

Barks, Coleman. 1995. *The essential Rumi*. San Francisco: HarperSanFrancisco.

Becker, Ernest. 1973. *The denial of death*. Glencoe, IL: Free Press.

Birren, James F. 1959. *Handbook of aging and the individual*. Chicago: Univ. of Chicago Press.

Buckley, Walter. 1967. *Sociology and modern systems theory*. Englewood Cliffs, NJ: Prentice-Hall.

Campbell, Joseph. 1972. *The hero with a thousand faces*. Princeton, NJ: Princeton Univ. Press.

Clark, Margaret, and Barbara Anderson. 1967. *Culture and aging*. Springfield, IL: Charles C Thomas.

Cohen, Gene D. 2000. *The creative age*. New York: Avon.

Cole, Thomas R. 1992. *The journey of life*. New York: Cambridge Univ. Press.

Cooley, Charles H. 1902. *Human nature and the social order*. New York: Scribners.

Csikszentmihalyi, Mihali. 1990. *Flow: The psychology of optimal experience*. New York: Harper & Row.

Dreher, Diane. 1996. *The Tao of personal leadership*. New York: HarperBusiness.

Erikson, Erik H. 1955. *Childhood and society*. New York: W. W. Norton.

———. 1963. *Childhood and society*, 2nd ed. New York: W. W. Norton.

———. 1980. *Identity and the life cycle*. New York: W. W. Norton.

Erikson, Erik H., Joan M. Erikson, and Helen Q. Kivnick. 1986. *Vital involvement in old age*. New York: W. W. Norton.

Erikson, Joan M. 1997. *The life cycle completed*. New York: W. W. Norton.

Fetzer Institute/National Institute on Aging Working Group. 2003. *Multidimensional measurement of religiousness/spirituality for use in health research*. Kalamazoo, MI: Fetzer Institute.

Fiske, Marjorie, and David A. Chiriboga. 1990. *Change and continuity in adult life*. San Francisco: Jossey-Bass.

Fowler, James W. 1981. *Stages of faith*. San Francisco: Harper & Row.

———. 1991. *Weaving the new creation: Stages of faith in the public church*. San Francisco: Harper & Row.

Frydman, Maurice. 1973. *I am that: Conversations with Sri Nisargadatta Maharaj*. Durham, NC: Acorn Press.

Gallup, George H., Jr. 2003. Americans' spiritual searches turn inward. GPNS Commentary, February 11. www.gallup.com.

———. 2003. Religious awakenings bolster Americans' faith. GPNS Commentary, January 14. www.gallup.com.

Gilley, Kay. 1997. *Leading from the heart.* Boston: Butterworth-Heinemann.

Girth, Hans, and C. Wright Mills. 1953. *Character and social structure: The psychology of social institutions.* New York: Harcourt, Brace & World.

Goffman, Erving. 1959. *The presentation of self in everyday life.* Garden City, NY: Doubleday.

Greenwald, Anthony. 1980. The totalitarian ego: Fabrication and revision of personal history. *American Psychologist* 35: 603–18.

Heidegger, Martin. [1959] 1966. *Discourse on thinking.* New York: Harper & Row.

Hellebrandt, Frances A. 1978. The senile dement in our midst. *Gerontologist* 18: 67–70.

Hillman, James. 1999. *The force of character and the lasting life.* New York: Random House.

Hixon, Lex. 1978. *Coming home: The experience of enlightenment in sacred traditions.* New York: Anchor Books.

Huxley, Aldous. 1944. *The perennial philosophy.* New York: Harper & Row.

James, William. [1905] 2005. *Varieties of religious experience: A study in human nature.* London: Longmans, Green & Co.

Jung, Carl G., and Aniela Jaffe. 1962. *Memories, dreams, and reflections.* London: Collins.

Kahn, Robert L., and Toni C. Antonucci. 1981. Convoys of social support: A life-course approach. In *Aging: Social change,* ed. S. B. Keisler et al., 383–405. New York: Academic Press.

Kastenbaum, Robert. 1993. Habituation: A key to lifespan development and aging? In *Encyclopedia of adult development,* ed. R. Kastenbaum, 195–200. Phoenix, AZ: Oryx Press.

———. 2004. *On our way: The final passage through life and death.* Berkeley, CA: Univ. of California Press.

Kelly, George A. 1955. *The psychology of personal constructs.* New York: W. W. Norton.

Koenig, Harold G. 1995. *Aging and God: Spiritual pathways to mental health in midlife and later years.* New York: Haworth Press.

Koenig, Harold G., Michael E. McCullough, and David B. Larson. 2001. *Handbook of religion and health.* New York: Oxford Univ. Press.

Levine, Stephen. 1982. *Who dies? An investigation of conscious living and conscious dying.* Garden City, NY: Doubleday.

Lindsay, Michael. 2000. Unchurched America has changed little in 20 years. Gallup News Service, March 28. www.gallup.com.

MacKinlay, Elizabeth. 2006. Spiritual care: Recognizing spiritual needs of older adults. *Journal of Religion, Spirituality, and Aging* 18 (2/3): 59–71.

Manheimer, Ronald J. 1999. *A map to the end of time: Wayfarings with friends and philosophers.* New York: W. W. Norton.

Markus, Hazel R., and A. Regula Herzog. 1991. The role of self concept in aging. *Annual Review of Gerontology and Geriatrics* 11: 110–43.

Markus, Hazel R., and Paula Nurius. 1986. Possible selves. *American Psychologist* 41: 954–69.

Maslow, Abraham. 1968. *Toward a psychology of being.* New York: Penguin.

Mead, George H. 1934. *Mind, self, and society.* Chicago: Univ. of Chicago Press.

Mitchell, Stephen. 1989. *The enlightened heart.* New York: Harper & Row.

———. 1991. *The enlightened mind.* New York: HarperCollins.

Moberg, David O., ed. 2001. *Aging and spirituality: Spiritual dimensions of aging theory, research, practice, and policy.* Binghamton, NY: Haworth Press.

Moody, Harry R., and David Carroll. 1997. *The five stages of the soul.* New York: Anchor Books.

Moody, Raymond A., Jr. 1977. *Life after life.* Toronto: Bantam.

Palmer, Parker J. 2004. *A hidden wholeness: The journey toward an undivided life.* San Francisco: Jossey-Bass.

Pargament, Kenneth I. 1997. *The psychology of religion and coping.* New York: Guilford.

Pascual-Leone, Juan. 1990. Reflections on life-span intelligence, consciousness, and ego development. In *Higher stages of human development,* ed. C. H. Alexander and E. J. Langer, 258–85. New York: Oxford Univ. Press.

Peacock, James R., and Margaret M. Paloma. 1991. Religiosity and life satisfaction across the life course. Paper presented at the Annual Meeting of the Society for the Scientific Study of Religion, November, Pittsburgh.

Prabhavananda, Swami, and Christopher Isherwood. 1944. *The song of God: Bhagavad-Gita.* New York: Penguin Group.

Radhakrishnan, S. 1989. *Indian philosophy.* London: Unwin Hyman.

Ram Dass. 1973. *Be here now.* San Cristobal, NM: Lama Foundation.

———. 1988. *Finding and exploring your spiritual path.* Los Angeles: Audio Renaissance Tapes.

———. 2000. *Still here: embracing aging, changing, and dying.* New York: Riverhead Books.

Ram Dass, and Paul Gorman. 1995. *How can I help? Stories and reflections on service.* New York: Alfred A. Knopf.

Ray, Ruth E., and Susan H. McFadden. 2001. The web and the quilt: Alternatives to the heroic journey toward spiritual development. *Journal of Adult Development* 8 (4): 201–11.

Riley, Matilda W., and Anne Foner, eds. 1968. *Aging and society.* Vol. 1: *An inventory of research findings.* New York: Russell Sage Foundation.

Rilke, Rainer Maria. [1929] 2002. *Letters to a young poet.* Mineola, NY: Dover.

Roof, Wade C. 1999. *Spiritual marketplace: Baby boomers and the remaking of American religion.* Princeton, NJ: Princeton Univ. Press.

Safransky, Sy. 1990. *Sunbeams: A book of quotations.* Berkeley, CA: North Atlantic Books.

Salthouse, Timothy H. 1982. *Adult cognition: An experimental psychology of human aging.* New York: Springer.

Schachter-Shalomi, Zalman, and Ronald S. Miller. 1995. *From age-ing to sage-ing: A profound new vision of growing older.* New York: Warner Books.

Settersten, Richard A., Jr. 1999. *Lives in time and place.* Amityville, NY: Baywood.

———. 2003. Propositions and controversies in life-course scholarship. In *Invitation to the life course,* ed. R. A. Settersten, Jr., 1–12. Amityville, NY: Baywood.

Smith, Huston. 2001. *Why religion matters: The fate of the human spirit in an age of disbelief.* New York: HarperCollins.

Surya Das. 1997. *Awakening the Buddha within.* New York: Broadway Books.

Tibbitts, Clark, ed. 1960. *Handbook of social gerontology.* Chicago: Univ. of Chicago Press.

Tillich, Paul. 1967. *Systematic theology: Three volumes in one.* Chicago: Univ. of Chicago Press.

Tolle, Eckhart. 1999. *The power of now.* Novato, CA: New World Library.

———. 2003. *Stillness speaks.* Novato, CA: New World Library.

Tornstam, Lars. 1994. Gerotranscendence: A theoretical and empirical exploration. In *Aging and the religious dimension,* ed. L. E. Thomas and S. A. Eisenhandler, 203–29. New York: Auburn House.

———. 2005. *Gerotranscendence: A developmental theory of positive aging.* New York: Springer.

Turner, Jonathan H. 1991. *The structure of sociological theory.* 5th ed. Belmont, CA: Wadsworth.

Vardey, Lucinda, ed. 1995. *God in all worlds: An anthology of contemporary spiritual writing.* New York: Pantheon Books.

Wade-Gayles, Gloria, and Ellen Finch. 1995. Three women's spiritual bonding on Sapelo Island. In *My soul is a witness: African-American women's spirituality,* ed. G. Wade-Gayles, 71–84. Boston: Beacon Press.

Walsh, Roger. 1999. *Essential spirituality: The seven central practices to awaken heart and mind.* New York: John Wiley & Sons.

Walsh, Roger, and F. Vaughan. 1993. On transpersonal definitions. *Journal of Transpersonal Psychology* 25 (2): 125–82.

Wegela, Karen K. 1996. *How to be a help instead of a nuisance.* Boston: Shambhala.

Wilber, Ken. 1983. *A sociable God: Toward a new understanding of religion.* Boston: Shambhala.

———. 2000. *Integral psychology.* Boston: Shambhala.

———. 2001. *Eye to eye: The quest for a new paradigm,* 3rd ed. Boston: Shambhala.

———. 2006. *Integral spirituality.* Boston: Integral Books.

Winseman, Albert L. 2003. Spiritual commitment by age and gender. Gallup News Service, March 11. www.gallup.com.

Wuthnow, Robert. 1998. *After heaven: Spirituality in America since the 1950s.* Berkeley, CA: Univ. of California Press.

Zinnbauer, Brian J., et al. 1997. Religion and spirituality: Unfuzzying the fuzzy. *Journal for the Scientific Study of Religion* 36 (4): 549–64.

Index

About the Author

Robert C. Atchley is an award-winning teacher, scholar, author, and mentor who, since 1985, has focused on the subject of how human beings develop spiritually and manifest spirituality in their lives. He has presented numerous lectures and workshops to a wide variety of audiences and has written more than a dozen articles on this subject for the general public. His knowledge of the subject comes from extensive interviews and research, participation in many working groups of researchers, writers, and lecturers focusing on spirituality, involvement in several organizations promoting "conscious aging" or spiritual growth, and his own thirty-year conscious spiritual journey.

In the mid-1970s, at age 35, Atchley began that journey. He read classic texts on spirituality from different spiritual traditions, attended workshops on meditation and spiritual development, went to India to study with the Indian sage Nisargadatta Maharaj, and spent several years teaching at Naropa University, which emphasizes contemplative education and is Buddhist-inspired. Since 1996 he has found spiritual community in Quaker Meetings.

In the 1980s, Atchley began teaching about spiritual development as part of his university course on adult development. He also began to include questions about spiritual life in his research interviews with middle-aged and older adults. In the 1990s, he published a series of articles on various aspects of spirituality and spiritual growth. He also became involved with the Omega Institute's series of programs on "conscious aging" and in the Spiritual Eldering Institute and the Sage-ing Guild. In addition to conducting many workshops on his own, he was co-presenter of workshops with Rabbi Zalman Schachter-Shalomi ("From Age-ing to Sage-ing") and with Ram Dass ("Conscious Aging"). Since 2000, he has published entries on spirituality for three encyclopedias.

Atchley is Distinguished Professor of Gerontology (emeritus) at Miami University, in Oxford, Ohio. He is author of more than twenty books and research monographs, including *Understanding American Society* (1970), *The Sociology of Retirement* (1976), *Aging: Continuity and Change* (1987), *Continuity and Adaptation in Aging: Creating Positive Experiences* (1999), and ten editions of his introductory gerontology text, *Social Forces and Aging* (2004).

He has received more than a dozen awards for his teaching, writing, and service, including the Distinguished Career Achievement Award from the Gerontological Society of America and the Benjamin Harrison Medallion, Miami University's highest honor given to a faculty member. He received the American Society on Aging's award for Distinguished Contribution to the Education of the Nation.